60 HIKES WITHIN 60 MILES

MADISON

Including DANE and Surrounding Counties

SECOND EDITION

Kevin Revolinski

MENASHA RIDGE PRESS
Birmingham, Alabama

60 Hikes Within 60 Miles: Madison

Copyright © 2015 by Kevin Revolinski
All rights reserved
Printed in the United States of America
Published by Menasha Ridge Press
Distributed by Publishers Group West
Second edition, first printing

Library of Congress Cataloging-in-Publication Data

Revolinski, Kevin.
  60 hikes within 60 miles, Madison : includes Dane and surrounding counties / Kevin Revolinski. —
Second Edition.
    pages cm
"Distributed by Publishers Group West"—T.p. verso.
Includes index.
  ISBN 978-1-63404-000-6 — ISBN 1-63404-000-7
  1. Hiking—Wisconsin—Madison Metropolitan Area—Guidebooks. 2. Trails—Wisconsin—Madison
Metropolitan Area—Guidebooks. 3. Madison Metropolitan Area (Wis.)—Guidebooks. I. Title. II. Title:
Sixty hikes within sixty miles.
  GV199.42.W62M34 2015
  796.5109775'83—dc23
                        2014047425

ISBN 978-1-63404-000-6; eISBN 978-1-63404-001-3

Cover design, cartography, and elevation profiles: Scott McGrew
Text design: Annie Long
Cover and interior photos by Kevin Revolinski, except where noted
Author photo by Preamtip Satasuk

 MENASHA RIDGE PRESS
An imprint of Keen Communications, LLC
2204 First Avenue South, Suite 102
Birmingham, AL 35233

Visit **menasharidge.com** for a complete listing of our books and for ordering information. Contact us at
our website, at **facebook.com/menasharidge**, or at **twitter.com/menasharidge** with questions or
comments. To find out more about who we are and what we're doing, visit our blog, **trekalong.com.**

DISCLAIMER

This book is meant only as a guide to select trails in the Madison area and does not guarantee hiker safety in any way—
you hike at your own risk. Neither Menasha Ridge Press nor Kevin Revolinski is liable for property loss or damage, per-
sonal injury, or death that result in any way from accessing or hiking the trails described in the following pages. Please be
aware that hikers have been injured in the Madison area. Be especially cautious when walking on or near boulders, steep
inclines, and drop-offs, and do not attempt to explore terrain that may be beyond your abilities. To help ensure an une-
ventful hike, please read carefully the introduction to this book, and perhaps get further safety information and guidance
from other sources. Familiarize yourself thoroughly with the areas you intend to visit before venturing out. Ask questions, and prepare for the unforeseen. Familiarize yourself with current weather reports, maps of the area you intend to
visit, and any relevant park regulations.

Table of Contents

Acknowledgments

I COULDN'T HAVE DONE this book without all the kind and generous contributions of so many people along the trail. Many of these thanks are more relevant to the first edition, but as this edition is built on the back of that one, it's only appropriate to leave them here, even if some of the folks have moved on to other parks or positions. Of course, there are hundreds of park managers, trail volunteers, land owners and donors, and fellow hikers, some of whom I've met and others who have done or continue to do great things to preserve the natural beauty of Wisconsin. But, in particular, I'd like to thank Sharon Kizer for a great starting list of recommendations. Thanks to Jen, Scott, and Evie Lynch for great suggestions for hikes for kids and a natural remedy for mosquito bites. The Ice Age Trail segments benefited from the information from Theresa Werner and Lorraine Lange, as well as Eric Sherman and Kevin Thusius of the Ice Age Park and Trail Foundation. Specifically for that great trail project, we all need to thank the private landowners who have been so kind as to allow us to tread upon portions of their property, as well as the many volunteers working hard to create the route.

I'm grateful to Danica for helping me sort out the labyrinth of an outdated map of a park full of uncharted trails. Cheers to Joel Green from the Department of Natural Resources and Sara Kehrli with Columbia County Parks for helping me find my way along some trails less traveled. More thanks go to Steve Johnston at New Glarus Woods State Park (and Badger State Trail), as well as David Borsecnik at the Department of Natural Resources (formerly at Lake Kegonsa State Park) and Chris James, Park Planner for Dane County. My gratitude to Molly and all the folks at Menasha Ridge Press, plus a big thanks to Johnny Molloy, mentor and all-around outdoor sensei, for continued advice and mental and tech support.

Further thanks to Mark and Janice Bauman for some update advice. And more thanks to Mary Michal and Sharon Fallon, who hiked the entire first edition and have kept me advised about some changes and trail-addition ideas, but most importantly, who shared their contagious enthusiasm for hiking. It makes all the work worth it.

I owe the continued health of my feet to Steve Schmitt of The Shoe Box in Black Earth, who was kind enough to donate a great pair of hiking boots to the cause when I did the first edition—and now they've survived a second. Still the best shoe store in Madison, though it isn't actually *in* Madison.

Thanks to Brian Babler for providing a backup when my GPS device seemed a little wonky; my cousin Renee Lajcak for some wildflower identification support; and Nicki Richmond, Kristin Abraham, and Mark Geske for some trail companionship. Thanks to my wife, Preamtip Satasuk, for the photos, much of the trip support, and for being a good sport when I found the road less traveled wasn't worth traveling and in fact was more akin to a bramble patch and not a good place to hike in shorts. My bad. Serious apologies for all the mosquito bites! And to my parents for finally giving up on trying to tell me I should be teaching. Their continued support means a ton to me.

Foreword

WELCOME TO MENASHA RIDGE PRESS'S *60 Hikes Within 60 Miles,* a series designed to provide hikers with the information they need to find and hike the very best trails surrounding metropolitan areas.

Our strategy is simple: First, find a hiker who knows the area and loves to hike. Second, ask that person to spend a year researching the most popular and very best trails around. And third, have that person describe each trail in terms of difficulty, scenery, condition, elevation change, and other categories of information that are important to hikers. "Pretend you've just completed a hike and met up with other hikers at the trailhead," we told each author. "Imagine their questions; be clear in your answers."

An experienced hiker and writer, Kevin Revolinski has selected 60 of the best hikes in and around the Madison metropolitan area. From the towering bluffs of Devil's Lake to an urban stroll around the capital, Revolinski provides hikers (and walkers) with a great variety of outings—all within roughly 60 miles of Madison.

You'll get more out of this book if you take a moment to read the Introduction, which explains how to read the trail listings. The "Topo Maps" section (page 5) will help you understand how useful topos are on a hike and also will tell you where to get them. And though this is a where-to, not a how-to, guide, readers who have not hiked extensively will find the Introduction of particular value.

As much for the opportunity to free the spirit as to free the body, let these hikes elevate you above the urban hurry.

All the best,

The Editors at Menasha Ridge Press

Preface

"I only went out for a walk and finally concluded to stay out till sundown, for going out, I found, was really going in." —John Muir

MADISON, THE SAYING GOES, is 76 square miles (an ever-changing number) surrounded by reality. The statement was meant as an attack on progressive-minded politics and perhaps the endless bickering that goes on here over what might be best for the community and Wisconsin at large. It's an impassioned population, to be sure. The reality that indeed surrounds us Madisonians, however, is some impressive land preservation, a great state park system, and ongoing restorations of forests, wetlands, prairie, savanna, and long-lost trout streams. Forward thinking has accomplished much in preserving the natural beauty of the area that might have otherwise been lost to reckless development.

So much of the region was once clear-cut for farming, wetlands were drained for the same, and trout streams were dammed for mill ponds. But a long line of environmentalists—including one-time resident and University of Wisconsin professor Aldo Leopold; land donors, such as the Frautschi family, Edna Taylor, and Edward T. Owen; and a small army of concerned citizens and activist groups—have all worked hard to keep Madison's relationship with the land and the environment harmonious. The city's Arboretum is considered a mainstay of our green space, a symbol of our love of natural beauty. Yet less than a century ago, hardly any of what we see today existed. Traces of the failed urban development known as the Lost City can still be found in the preserve's soggy soil. From one park to the next, efforts are being made to restore prairies to the way they were before European settlers arrived. Oak savanna and forests have also made their comebacks.

The state of Wisconsin, the city of Madison, and all the neighboring communities, from the Dells to Janesville and from Dodgeville to Delafield, have put public resources into various trail and park projects. But more important than anything has been the contribution of the thousands of volunteers who maintain trails, compile maps, run websites, and organize events. The money of private donors and the easements granted by private landowners are what make something as magnificent and massive as the Ice Age National Scenic Trail possible. Much of what I've hiked on the IAT is someone's backyard or overgrown farmland.

In terms of hiking trails, there is something for everyone here. Treks range from easy strolls not far from home, such as Picnic Point along Lake Mendota, to the challenging 18-mile hike of the Ice Age Trail segment that climbs both 500-foot bluffs at Devil's Lake State Park. Within a 60-mile radius, you can find migrating birds and wetlands in Horicon Marsh, deer and prairie flowers in New Glarus Woods, trout flitting in the shadows of Rowan Creek, and the marks of the last advance of the glaciers in Kettle Moraine State Forest.

History hiked these trails as well, and you can visit the tragic battlegrounds of Sauk warrior Black Hawk, where he made a stand that allowed his people to escape, albeit temporarily, across the Wisconsin River in 1832. Find enchantment in the mysterious archaeological remains at Aztalan or the many Native American effigy mounds in several of the parks, or discover the remains of Civilian Conservation Corps projects or pioneer settlements.

Those fascinated by geology should be adequately impressed by the sandstone rock outcrops of Green, Rock, Dane, Columbia, and Sauk counties, which date to between 460 million and 550 million years ago. All of that looks a bit recent, however, when compared to the quartzite of the Baraboo Hills and Devil's Lake bluffs in Sauk County, which is said to be 1.6 billion years old.

Southern Wisconsin is neither the remote woods of Appalachia nor the secluded mountains of the West, to be sure. But the reestablishment of the ecosystems of yesteryear and the outstanding state and county park systems provide places that seem a hundred miles away from the last human outpost, and yet all lie within an hour of your front door.

City of Madison

In 1908, John Olin and the members of the Madison Park and Pleasure Drive Association brought in landscape architect John Nolen, who in turn set out much of the urban plan for parks in the city of Madison and even provided the foundations for the state park system. Nolen believed that "simple recreation in the open air amid beautiful surroundings contributes to physical and moral health, to a saner and happier life." Thanks to him and some like-minded Madisonians, we have a variety of excellent parks, including the Arboretum, which offers several escapes from the city in the very *heart* of the city along the shores of Lake Wingra.

The Ho Chunk tribe referred to the Madison area as Dejope, meaning "four lakes." The lakes define Madison, and the hike to Picnic Point is a classic, simply synonymous with the Madison experience and one of the best ways to see Lake Mendota and the Capitol. Olin Park and Turville Point see the dome from the Lake Monona side. The Yahara River and its watershed feed the lakes and create wetlands, such as Cherokee Marsh and Token Creek, which provide good wildlife viewing and easy strolls along grassy paths and boardwalks.

University Professor Edward T. Owen feared that reckless urban development would spoil the natural beauty of Madison. He did much to develop pleasure drives in the late 19th century, and he and his colleagues John Olin and Edward Hammersley donated land for that purpose. Now Owen's former summer retreat is a west-side conservation park, prime for birders and offering trails that make the surrounding cityscape seem nonexistent. Edna Taylor Conservation Park and the Aldo Leopold Nature Center do the same for the east side of town.

The Meccas

KETTLE MORAINE STATE FOREST

The most recent period of the Ice Age is known as the Wisconsin Glaciation. It came to its dwindling end in a jagged line across the state about 10,000 years ago. Thanks to the land-altering efforts of an ice sheet that was as much as a mile thick in some places, there is no better place to see the dramatic effects of continental glaciers than in Wisconsin. Two massive lobes of glacial ice left behind two ridges approximately 120 miles long in the southeastern part of the state. Melting ice buried within glacial deposits left kettlelike depressions that have since been overgrown with hardwood forests and, in some cases, filled in with bogs. The very ground beneath your feet is strewn with sand and broken rock, some of which may have originated all the way back in Canada.

THE ICE AGE TRAIL

This is a project in development. The ultimate goal is a 1,000-mile national scenic trail that roughly follows the terminal edge of the last glaciation. The trails are often rugged and secluded and tend to be some of the more challenging hikes. It is possible to camp along parts of the trail, and many hikers set out to hike it all either in increments or at a go. Roadways and a network of urban streets connect the wilderness segments, but many of the segments in this book are good out-and-back or one-way treks that can be done in as little as an hour or as much as an entire day.

DEVIL'S LAKE STATE PARK

This is arguably the most popular of the area state parks. Nothing rivals the views from atop the two 500-foot rocky bluffs, other than perhaps Gibraltar Rock State Natural Area. Though steep at times, the trails along the cliffs are nicely laid out with stone steps and asphalt. Between the two bluffs lies the lake. A whole network of trails explores the woods and prairies beyond the East Bluff, and great facilities make the park ideal for camping or having a swim at one of two beaches. The tumbled quartzite talus along the slopes and the rock formations and glacial moraines will impress as well.

THE "DRIFTLESS" AREA

The stopping line of the last glaciers passes right through this book's territory; crossing from Ice Age country, you enter the Driftless Area, characterized by river valleys, rolling hills, caves, springs, and sinkholes. No natural lakes occur here as no glacial debris or "drift" was left to block springs and streams. At Blue Mound State Park, you can find an abundance of springwater bubbling its way down the rocky terrain in the forest. The view from the untouched bluff reaches to a far horizon, and the mound itself is visible all the way back in Madison. Governor Dodge State Park has a hike through a sandstone canyon and around two lakes formed from the damming of a spring creek that should not be missed.

60 Hikes by Category

Hike Categories

• distance (mi)	• wheelchair/	• scenic views	• dog-friendly
• difficulty*	stroller-friendly	• kid-friendly	• running

* Difficulty: **E** = easy, **M** = moderate, **S** = strenuous

REGION Hike Number/Hike Name	page	distance (mi)	difficulty	wheelchair/ stroller-friendly	scenic views	kid-friendly	dog-friendly	running
MADISON METRO								
1 Arboretum: Greene Prairie	18	2.6	E–M			✓		
2 Arboretum: Wingra Marsh	22	1.6	E			✓		✓
3 Arboretum: Wingra Woods	26	2.4	E–M			✓		
4 Capital City State Trail: E-Way Segment	31	8–16	E	✓			✓	✓
5 Cherokee Marsh North	35	2	E–M					
6 Cherokee Marsh South	39	3	E–M					
7 Edna Taylor Conservation Park	45	3.1	E			✓		
8 Elver Park	50	3.4	E–M					✓
9 Lewis Nine Springs E-Way Trail	54	5.4	E			✓		
10 Madison Capitol and Downtown	59	3	E	✓			✓	
11 Olin Park and Turville Point Conservation Park	64	2	E					
12 Owen Conservation Park	68	1.5	E–M					✓
13 Pheasant Branch Conservancy	72	up to 7.6	E–M	✓	✓	✓	✓	✓
14 Picnic Point	77	8	E–M	portions	✓	✓		✓
15 Pope Farm Park	82	2.5	E–M			✓		
16 Tenney Park to Schenk's Corners	87	3.9	E	✓			✓	
17 Token Creek	92	3.7	E	portions			✓	
18 Tom George Greenway	97	2.2	E–M			✓		✓

REGION Hike Number/Hike Name		page	distance (mi)	difficulty	wheelchair/ stroller-friendly	scenic views	kid-friendly	dog-friendly	running
NORTHWEST									
19	Black Hawk Unit: Lower Wisconsin State Riverway	104	9.5	E–D		✓	✓	✓	
20	Devil's Lake State Park: East Bluff	109	5.6	D		✓	✓	✓	
21	Devil's Lake State Park: West Bluff	113	2.7	M–D		✓		✓	
22	Gibraltar Rock State Natural Area	117	1.4–2.8	M–D		✓		✓	
23	Governor Nelson State Park	121	3.9	E–M	portions		✓		
24	Ice Age Trail: Cross Plains Segment	126	2.8	E–M		✓	✓	✓	
25	Ice Age Trail: Devil's Lake Segment	130	up to 21.1	M–D		✓	✓		
26	Ice Age Trail: Groves-Pertzborn Segment	136	2.6	M–D			✓	✓	
27	Ice Age Trail: Lodi Marsh Segment	140	7.8	M				✓	
28	Ice Age Trail: Table Bluff Segment	144	5	M–D		✓		✓	
29	Indian Lake County Park	149	4.7	E–M			✓		
30	Mirror Lake State Park	154	3.3–4.3	E–M	✓	✓	✓	✓	
31	Natural Bridge State Park	159	2.4	M–D				✓	
32	Pewit's Nest	164	0.9	M–D		✓			
33	Rocky Arbor State Park	169	1.1	M–D			✓	✓	
34	Rowan Creek Trail	173	2.8	E			✓	✓	
35	Swan Lake State Wildlife Area	177	3.8	M			✓	✓	
SOUTHWEST									
36	Badger State Trail	184	18	E	✓			✓	
37	Blue Mound State Park	189	up to 5.6	E–D		✓	✓	✓	
38	Cadiz Springs State Recreation Area	194	4.2	E			✓	✓	
39	Donald County Park	198	4.5	M			✓	✓	
40	Governor Dodge State Park: Lost Canyon Trail	202	8.8	M		x	✓	✓	

REGION Hike Number/Hike Name	page	distance (mi)	difficulty	wheelchair/ stroller-friendly	scenic views	kid-friendly	dog-friendly	running
SOUTHWEST *(continued)*								
41 Governor Dodge State Park: White Oak Trail	206	4.3	M		✓			
42 Ice Age Trail: Brooklyn Wildlife Segment	210	6.8	M–D				✓	
43 Ice Age Trail: Montrose Segment	215	4.6	M		✓		✓	
44 Ice Age Trail: Verona Segment	219	up to 12.6	E–M				✓	
45 Magnolia Bluff Park	223	2.4	M		✓		✓	
46 New Glarus Woods State Park	227	3.8	M			✓	✓	
47 Stewart County Park	232	3.6	M				✓	
48 Yellowstone Lake State Park	237	9.4	E–M		✓	✓	✓	
NORTHEAST								
49 Horicon Marsh State Wildlife Area	244	4.7	E					
50 Horicon National Wildlife Refuge	248	4.3	E	✓			✓	
SOUTHEAST								
51 Aztalan State Park	254	1.8	E–M	✓		✓	✓	
52 CamRock Park: Area 2	259	2.2	E				✓	
53 Glacial Drumlin State Trail	264	13.2	E	✓				
54 Ice Age Trail: Devil's Staircase Segment	268	2.8–5.6	M–D		✓			
55 Ice Age Trail: Whitewater Lake Segment	272	8.9	M–D				✓	
56 Kettle Moraine State Forest: John Muir Trail	276	9.5	M–D				✓	
57 Kettle Moraine State Forest: Lapham Peak Unit	280	6.9	M–D				✓	
58 Kettle Moraine State Forest: Nordic Trails	285	up to 9.1	E–D				✓	
59 Kettle Moraine State Forest: ScuppernongTrail	289	5.4	E–M				✓	
60 Lake Kegonsa State Park	293	5.3	E	✓		✓	✓	✓

More Hike Categories

- streams, rivers, lakes, and wetlands
- busy
- solitude
- wildflowers
- wildlife
- bird-watching
- historic interest

REGION Hike Number/Hike Name	page	streams, rivers, lakes, and wetlands	busy	solitude	wildflowers	wildlife	bird-watching	historic interest
MADISON METRO								
1 Arboretum: Greene Prairie	18				✓		✓	
2 Arboretum: Wingra Marsh	22	✓						
3 Arboretum: Wingra Woods	26						✓	
4 Capital City State Trail: E-Way Segment	31		✓		✓			
5 Cherokee Marsh North	35		✓				✓	
6 Cherokee Marsh South	39		✓				✓	
7 Edna Taylor Conservation Park	45		✓		✓	✓	✓	
8 Elver Park	50	✓						
9 Lewis Nine Springs E-Way Trail	54		✓		✓	✓		
10 Madison Capitol and Downtown	59	✓	✓					✓
11 Olin Park and Turville Point Conservation Park	64		✓					
12 Owen Conservation Park	68				✓			✓
13 Pheasant Branch Conservancy	72	✓						
14 Picnic Point	77	✓	✓					
15 Pope Farm Park	82		✓					
16 Tenney Park to Schenk's Corners	87							✓
17 Token Creek	92	✓					✓	
18 Tom George Greenway	97			✓				
NORTHWEST								
19 Black Hawk Unit: Lower Wisconsin State Riverway	104					✓	✓	✓
20 Devil's Lake State Park: East Bluff	109				✓		✓	
21 Devil's Lake State Park: West Bluff	113				✓		✓	
22 Gibraltar Rock State Natural Area	117						✓	

REGION Hike Number/Hike Name	page	streams, rivers, lakes, and wetlands	busy	solitude	wildflowers	wildlife	bird-watching	historic interest
NORTHWEST *(continued)*								
23 Governor Nelson State Park	121				✓	✓		
24 Ice Age Trail: Cross Plains Segment	126				✓			
25 Ice Age Trail: Devil's Lake Segment	130	✓				✓		
26 Ice Age Trail: Groves-Pertzborn Segment	136			✓		✓		
27 Ice Age Trail: Lodi Marsh Segment	140	✓		✓		✓		
28 Ice Age Trail: Table Bluff Segment	144			✓	✓	✓		
29 Indian Lake County Park	149	✓				✓		✓
30 Mirror Lake State Park	154	✓		✓		✓		
31 Natural Bridge State Park	159					✓		✓
32 Pewit's Nest	164	✓						
33 Rocky Arbor State Park	169							
34 Rowan Creek Trail	173	✓						
35 Swan Lake State Wildlife Area	177	✓		✓		✓		
SOUTHWEST								
36 Badger State Trail	184		✓					
37 Blue Mound State Park	189							
38 Cadiz Springs State Recreation Area	194	✓						
39 Donald County Park	198	✓		✓				
40 Governor Dodge State Park: Lost Canyon Trail	202	✓				✓		
41 Governor Dodge State Park: White Oak Trail	206	✓				✓		
42 Ice Age Trail: Brooklyn Wildlife Segment	210			✓	✓	✓		
43 Ice Age Trail: Montrose Segment	215			✓	✓	✓		
44 Ice Age Trail: Verona Segment	219	✓						
45 Magnolia Bluff Park	223							
46 New Glarus Woods State Park	227					✓		
47 Stewart County Park	232			✓	✓	✓	✓	

REGION Hike Number/Hike Name	page	streams, rivers, lakes, and wetlands	busy	solitude	wildflowers	wildlife	bird-watching	historic interest
SOUTHWEST *(continued)*								
48 Yellowstone Lake State Park	237	✓					✓	✓	
NORTHEAST								
49 Horicon Marsh State Wildlife Area	244	✓						✓	
50 Horicon National Wildlife Refuge	248	✓						✓	
SOUTHEAST								
51 Aztalan State Park	254	✓							✓
52 CamRock Park: Area 2	259	✓							
53 Glacial Drumlin State Trail	264		✓						
54 Ice Age Trail: Devil's Staircase Segment	268	✓						✓	
55 Ice Age Trail: Whitewater Lake Segment	272	✓			✓		✓		
56 Kettle Moraine State Forest: John Muir Trail	276								
57 Kettle Moraine State Forest: Lapham Peak Unit	280								
58 Kettle Moraine State Forest: Nordic Trails	285					✓	✓	✓	
59 Kettle Moraine State Forest: ScuppernongTrail	289								
60 Lake Kegonsa State Park	293	✓				✓		✓	

Arboretum: Wingra Marsh (see page 22)

Introduction

How to Use This Guidebook

OVERVIEW MAP, OVERVIEW-MAP KEY, AND MAP LEGEND

USE THE OVERVIEW MAP on the inside front cover to assess the general locations of each hike's primary trailhead. Each hike's number appears on the overview map, on the map key facing the overview map, and in the table of contents. As you flip through the book, a hike's full profile is easy to locate by watching for the hike number at the top of each page. The book is organized by region, as indicated in the table of contents. A map legend that details the symbols found on trail maps appears on the inside back cover.

REGIONAL MAPS

The book is divided into regions. Prefacing each regional section is an overview map of that region. The regional map provides more detail than the overview map, bringing you closer to the hike.

GPS INFORMATION

To produce the highly accurate maps in this book, I used a handheld GPS unit to gather data while hiking each route, and then I sent that data to Menasha Ridge Press's expert cartographers. Provided for each hike profile, the GPS coordinates—the intersection of latitude (north) and longitude (west)—will orient you from the trailhead. In some cases, you can park within viewing distance of a trailhead. Other hiking routes require a short walk to the trailhead from a parking area.

The latitude–longitude grid system is likely quite familiar to you, but here's a refresher, pertinent to visualizing the coordinates:

Imaginary lines of latitude—called *parallels* and approximately 69 miles apart from each other—run horizontally around the globe. The equator is established to be 0°, and each parallel is indicated by degrees from the equator: up to 90°N at the North Pole, and down to 90°S at the South Pole.

Imaginary lines of longitude—called *meridians*—run perpendicular to lines of latitude and are likewise indicated by degrees. Starting from 0° at the Prime Meridian in Greenwich, England, they continue to the east and west until they meet 180° later at the International Date Line in the Pacific Ocean. At the equator, longitude lines are also approximately 69 miles apart, but that distance narrows as the meridians converge toward the North and South Poles.

In this book, latitude and longitude are given in degrees, minutes, and seconds. For example, the coordinates for Hike 1, Arboretum: Greene Prairie (page 18), are as follows:

N43° 02' 2.99" W89° 26' 36.24".

For more on GPS technology, visit **usgs.gov.**

Hike Profiles

Each hike contains seven or eight key items: an "In Brief" description of the trail, a key at-a-glance information box, directions to the trail, GPS coordinates, a trail map, an elevation profile (if the elevation gain/loss exceeds 100 feet), a trail description, and notes on things to see and do nearby. Combined, the maps and information provide a clear method to assess each trail from the comfort of your favorite reading chair.

TRAIL MAPS

A detailed map of each hike's route appears with its profile. On each of these maps, symbols indicate the trailhead, the complete route, significant features, facilities, and topographic landmarks, such as creeks, overlooks, and peaks.

ELEVATION PROFILES

Each hike with an elevation gain/loss of more than 100 feet contains a detailed elevation profile that corresponds directly to the trail map. This graphical element provides a quick look at the trail from the side, enabling you to visualize how the trail rises and falls. On the diagram's vertical axis, or height scale, the number of feet indicated between each tick mark lets you visualize the climb. To avoid making flat hikes look steep and steep hikes appear flat, varying height scales provide an accurate image of each hike's climbing challenge. Elevation profiles for loop hikes show total distance; those for out-and-back hikes show only one-way distance.

IN BRIEF

This is a "taste of the trail." Think of this section as a snapshot focused on the historical landmarks, beautiful vistas, and other sights you might encounter on the hike.

KEY AT-A-GLANCE INFORMATION

The information in the key at-a-glance boxes gives you a quick idea of the statistics and specifics of each hike.

LENGTH & CONFIGURATION The length of the trail from start to finish (total distance traveled). There may be options to shorten or extend the hikes, but the mileage corresponds to the described hike. Consult the hike description to help decide how to customize the hike for your ability or time constraints. This line also provides a description of what the trail might look like from overhead. Trails can be loops, out-and-backs (trails on which one enters and leaves along the same path), figure eights, or a combination of shapes.

DIFFICULTY The degree of effort an average hiker should expect on a given hike. For simplicity, the trails are rated as easy, moderate, or difficult.

SCENERY A short summary of the attractions offered by the hike and what to expect in terms of plant life, wildlife, natural wonders, and historic features.

EXPOSURE A quick check of how much sun you can expect on your shoulders during the hike.

TRAFFIC Indicates how busy the trail might be on an average day. Trail traffic, of course, varies from day to day and season to season. Weekend days typically see the most visitors. Other trail users that you might encounter on the trail are also noted here.

TRAIL SURFACE Indicates whether the trail surface is paved, rocky, gravel, dirt, boardwalk, or a mixture of elements.

HIKING TIME The length of time it takes to hike the trail. A slow but steady hiker will average 2–3 miles per hour, depending on the terrain.

DRIVING DISTANCE Indicates expected distance from an easily identified point.

ACCESS Indicates whether a hike can be enjoyed year-round or only during certain times of the year.

WHEELCHAIR ACCESSIBILITY What to expect in terms of access to trail and facilities.

MAPS A list of maps that show the topography of the trail, including Green Trails Maps and USGS topo maps.

FACILITIES What to expect in terms of restrooms, water, and other amenities at the trailhead or nearby.

CONTACT Websites and phone numbers, where applicable, for up-to-date information on trail conditions.

COMMENTS Information about dog rules, fees, and other handy tips.

Note: Trails in the state parks often require a permit for parking: A day pass is $7, and the annual sticker is $25. If you plan to hike or visit the parks frequently each year, it is worth buying the annual sticker. Stickers can be purchased at state park offices or Department of Natural Resources service centers; they are also available online through the Wisconsin Department of Natural Resources website (**dnr.wi.gov/topic/parks/admission.html**). City and county parks typically do not require any permits or parking fees.

GPS TRAILHEAD COORDINATES

These may be used, in conjunction with the directions to the trail (below), to ascertain exactly where the trailhead is.

DIRECTIONS

Used in conjunction with the overview map, the driving directions will help you locate each trailhead. Once at the trailhead, park only in designated areas.

DESCRIPTION

The trail description is the heart of each hike. Here, the author provides a summary of the trail's essence and highlights any special traits the hike has to offer. The route is clearly outlined, including landmarks, side trips, and possible alternate routes along the way. Ultimately, the hike description will help you choose which hikes are best for you.

NEARBY ACTIVITIES

Look here for information on nearby activities or points of interest. This includes nearby parks, museums, restaurants, or even a brewpub where you can get a well-deserved beer after a long hike.

Weather

Madison enjoys all four seasons. Flowers and trees start to bloom by late April on into June. Colors change from late September through October, and snow might start to stick by the end of November. While each season brings exciting changes in the flora and fauna, the temperatures don't always abide by the start dates. Be prepared for a wide range of temperatures and conditions, regardless of the season. Winters typically offer temperatures well below freezing and moderate snowfall with the occasional blizzard; summers go to the other extreme with high humidity and temperatures often reaching the upper 80s to 90s. The average annual precipitation is 37 inches, and it comes in a rather even distribution throughout the year. Typically, June is the wettest month.

AVERAGE TEMPERATURE BY MONTH					
	JAN	**FEB**	**MAR**	**APR**	**MAY**	**JUN**
High	26°F	31°F	43°F	57°F	70°F	78°F
Low	10°F	14°F	25°F	35°F	46°F	56°F
	JUL	**AUG**	**SEP**	**OCT**	**NOV**	**DEC**
High	82°F	79°F	71°F	60°F	43°F	30°F
Low	61°F	59°F	50°F	39°F	28°F	16°F

Topo Maps

The maps in this book have been produced with great care and the assistance of a GPS unit. When used with the route directions present in each profile, the maps are sufficient to direct you to the trail and guide you on it. However, you will find superior detail and valuable information in the U.S. Geological Survey's (USGS) 7.5-minute series topographic maps.

Topo maps are available online in many locations. At **MyTopo.com,** for example, you can view and print topos of the entire United States free of charge. Online services, such as **Trails.com,** charge annual fees for additional features like shaded relief, which makes the topography stand out more. If you expect to print out many topo maps each year, it might be worth paying for shaded-relief topo maps. The downside to USGS topos is that most of them are outdated, having been created 20–30 years ago. But they still provide excellent topographic detail. Of course, **Google Earth (earth.google.com)** does away with topo maps and their inaccuracies—replacing them with satellite imagery and its inaccuracies. Regardless, what one lacks, the other augments. Google Earth is an excellent tool, whether you have difficulty with topos or not.

If you're new to hiking, you might be wondering, "What's a topographic map?" In short, a topo indicates not only linear distance but also elevation, using contour lines. Contour lines spread across the map like dozens of intricate spiderwebs. Each line represents a particular elevation; at the base of each topo, a contour's interval designation is given. If the contour interval is 20 feet, then the distance between each contour line is 20 feet. Follow five contour lines up on the same map, and the elevation has increased by 100 feet.

Let's assume that the 7.5-minute series topo reads "Contour Interval 40 feet," that the short trail we'll be hiking is 2 inches in length on the map, and that it crosses five contour lines from beginning to end. What do we know? Well, because the linear scale of this series is 2,000 feet to the inch (roughly 2.75 inches representing 1 mile), we know our trail is approximately 0.8-mile long (2 inches are 4,000 feet). But we also know we'll be climbing or descending 200 vertical feet (five contour lines are 40 feet each) over that distance. And the elevation designations written on occasional contour lines will tell us if we're heading up or down.

In addition to the outdoor shops listed in Appendix A, you'll find topos at major universities and some public libraries, where you might try photocopying what you need. But if you want your own and can't find them locally, visit **nationalmap.gov** or **store.usgs.gov.**

Water

How much is enough? Well, one simple physiological fact should convince you to err on the side of excess when deciding how much water to pack: A hiker working hard in 90°

heat needs approximately 10 quarts of fluid per day. That's 2.5 gallons—12 large water bottles or 16 small ones. In other words, pack along one or two bottles even for short hikes.

Some hikers and backpackers hit the trail prepared to purify water found along the route. This method, while less dangerous than drinking it untreated, comes with risks. Purifiers with ceramic filters are the safest. Many hikers pack along the slightly distasteful tetraglycine-hydroperiodide tablets to debug water (sold under the names Potable Aqua, Coughlan's, and others).

Probably the most common waterborne "bug" that hikers face is *Giardia,* which may not hit until one to four weeks after ingestion. It will have you living in the bathroom, passing noxious rotten-egg gas, vomiting, and shivering with chills. Other parasites to worry about include *E. coli* and *Cryptosporidium,* both of which are harder to kill than *Giardia.*

For most people, the pleasures of hiking make carrying water a relatively minor price to pay to remain healthy. If you're tempted to drink "found water," do so only if you understand the risks involved. Better yet, hydrate prior to your hike, carry (and drink) 6 ounces of water for every mile you plan to hike, and hydrate after the hike.

Clothing

There is a wide variety of clothing from which to choose. Basically, use common sense and be prepared for anything. If all you have are cotton clothes when a sudden rainstorm comes along, you'll be miserable, especially in cooler weather. It's a good idea to carry along a light wool sweater or some type of synthetic apparel (polypropylene, Capilene, Thermax, etc.) as well as a hat.

Be aware of the weather forecast and its tendency to be wrong. Always carry raingear. Thunderstorms can come on suddenly in the summer. Keep in mind that rainy days are as much a part of nature as those idyllic ones you desire. Besides, rainy days really cut down on the crowds. With appropriate raingear, a normally crowded trail can be a wonderful place of solitude. Do, however, remain aware of the dangers of lightning strikes.

Footwear is another concern. Though tennis shoes may be appropriate for paved areas, many trails are rocky and rough; tennis shoes may not offer enough support. Waterproofed or not, boots should be your footwear of choice. Sport sandals are more popular than ever, but these leave much of your foot exposed, leaving you vulnerable to hazardous plants and thorns or the occasional piece of glass.

The 10 Essentials

One of the first rules of hiking is to be prepared for anything. The simplest way to be prepared is to carry the "10 Essentials." In addition to carrying the items listed below, you need to know how to use them, especially navigational items. Always consider worst-case scenarios such as getting lost, hiking back in the dark, broken gear (for example, a broken hip strap on your pack or a plugged water filter), a twisted ankle, or a brutal thunderstorm. The items listed below don't cost a lot of money, don't take up much room in a pack, and don't weigh much, but they might just save your life.

- *Water:* durable bottles and water treatment, such as iodine or a filter
- *Map:* preferably a topo map and a trail map with a route description
- *Compass:* a high-quality compass (most smartphones have this feature)
- *First-aid kit:* a good-quality kit, including first-aid instructions
- *Knife:* preferably a multitool device with pliers
- *Light:* flashlight or headlamp with extra bulbs and batteries
- *Fire:* windproof matches or lighter and fire starter
- *Extra food:* You should always have food in your pack when you've finished hiking.
- *Extra clothes:* rain protection, warm layers, gloves, warm hat
- *Sun protection:* sunglasses, lip balm, sunblock, sun hat

First-Aid Kit

A typical first-aid kit may contain more items than you might think necessary. These are just the basics. Prepackaged kits in waterproof bags (Atwater Carey and Adventure Medical make a variety of kits) are available. Even though there are quite a few items listed here, they pack down into a small space:

- Ace bandages or Spenco joint wraps
- Antibiotic ointment (Neosporin or the generic equivalent)
- Aspirin or acetaminophen
- Band-Aids
- Benadryl or the generic equivalent diphenhydramine (in case of allergic reactions)
- Butterfly-closure bandages
- Epinephrine in a prefilled syringe (for people known to have severe allergic reactions to such things as bee stings)
- Gauze (one roll and a half dozen 4-by-4-inch pads)
- Hydrogen peroxide or iodine
- Insect repellent
- Matches or pocket lighter
- Moleskin/Spenco 2nd Skin
- Sunscreen
- Whistle (more effective in signaling rescuers than your voice)

Hiking with Children

No one is too young for a hike in the outdoors. Be mindful, though. Flat, short, and shaded trails are best with an infant. Toddlers who have not quite mastered walking can still tag along, riding on an adult's back in a child carrier. Use common sense to judge a child's capacity to hike a particular trail, and always anticipate that the child will tire quickly and need to be carried.

When packing for the hike, remember the child's needs as well as your own. Make sure children are adequately clothed for the weather, have proper shoes, and are protected from the sun with sunscreen. Kids dehydrate quickly, so make sure you have plenty of water for everyone. To assist you with determining which trails are suitable for children, a list of hike recommendations for children is provided on pages xii–xiv.

Many of Wisconsin's state parks participate in the Junior Rangers/Wisconsin Explorers Program, an environmental education activity program for children and their parents. Activity booklets for Junior Rangers (grades K–3) or Wisconsin Explorers (grades 4 and up) are available at most park offices. When at least half of the activities in the booklet are completed, the child is awarded a patch and certificate, available either from the park office or by mail. State parks also offer collectible cards for flora and fauna.

The outdoor store REI offers a variety of great information on their website. Go to **rei. com,** click on Learn, and then click on Family Adventure Program. Select Wisconsin and then Madison. You'll find region-specific information, day-hiking checklists, and more.

General Safety

No doubt, potentially dangerous situations can occur outdoors, but, as long as you use sound judgment and prepare yourself before hitting the trail, you'll be much safer in the woods than in most urban areas of the country. Here are a few tips to make your trip safer and easier.

➢ *Be careful at overlooks.* While these areas may provide spectacular views, they are potentially hazardous. Stay back from the edge of outcrops and be absolutely sure of your footing; a misstep can mean a nasty and possibly fatal fall. Many of the outcrops in this book are in areas of abundant sandstone, and a slippery fine layer of sand may go unnoticed.

➢ *Standing dead trees and storm-damaged living trees pose a real hazard* to hikers and tent campers. These trees may have loose or broken limbs that could fall at any time. When choosing a spot to rest or a backcountry campsite, look up. While hiking this guide, a very large portion of an unhealthy tree fell not 40 feet from me as I passed. Such an event is unlikely and a case of bad timing but something to be aware of.

➢ *Take along your brain.* A cool, calculating mind is the single most important piece of equipment you'll ever need on the trail. Think before you act. Watch your step. Plan ahead. Avoiding accidents before they happen is the best recipe for a rewarding and relaxing hike.

> ➢ *Ask questions.* Park employees are there to help. It's a lot easier to gain advice beforehand and avoid a mishap away from civilization when it's too late to amend an error. Use your head out there, and treat the place as if it were your own backyard.

> ➢ *Always tell at least two "keepers"* (people you trust) where you are hiking, and text them at regular intervals to let them know of your progress. Why two? One will likely get distracted and forget they are supposed to be your safety net.

> ➢ *Never tell someone you meet on the trail that you are hiking alone.* Always be hiking with "someone who is a little ahead of you or is catching up."

> ➢ *Know when sundown and nightfall occur,* and plan to be out of the woods prior to nightfall. If you get delayed and you are hiking in the dark, go slowly and use your flashlight intermittently to see the trail.

Animal and Plant Hazards

TICKS

Ticks like to hang out in the brush that grows along trails. Their numbers seem to explode in the hot summer months, but you should be tick-aware during all months of the year. Ticks, which are arthropods and not insects, need a host to feast on in order to reproduce. The ticks that light onto you while hiking will be very small, sometimes so tiny that you won't be able to spot them. The two primary varieties, deer ticks and dog ticks, both need a few hours of actual attachment before they can transmit any disease they may harbor. Ticks may settle in shoes, socks, and hats and may take several hours to actually latch on. The best strategy is to visually check every half-hour or so while hiking, do a thorough check before you get in the car, and then, when you take a posthike shower, do an even more thorough check of your entire body. Also, throw clothes into the dryer for 10 minutes when you get home, and be sure to check your pet for any hitchhikers. Ticks that haven't attached are easily removed but not easily killed. If you pick off a tick in the woods, just toss it aside. If you find one on your body at home, dispatch it and then send it down the toilet. For ticks that have embedded, removal with tweezers is best.

The deer tick is the culprit behind Lyme disease and, unfortunately, it is the smaller of the two ticks, as small as a poppy seed. Experts advocate abundant repellent containing permethrin on footwear and pant legs, because the nymphal-stage deer tick often lurks in dead leaves and ticks rarely climb higher than 18–24 inches off the ground. They can grab on to your shoes and are quite quick to climb up. Get more information from the American Lyme Disease Foundation at **aldf.com.**

MOSQUITOES

Although it's not a common occurrence, individuals can become infected with the West Nile virus by being bitten by an infected mosquito. Culex mosquitoes, the primary variety that can transmit West Nile virus to humans, thrive in urban rather than natural areas. They lay their eggs in stagnant water and can breed in standing water that remains for more than five days. Most people infected with West Nile virus have no symptoms of illness, but some may become ill, usually 3–15 days after being bitten.

In the Madison area, the risk period runs from mid-June to early October, with August and September being the riskiest months. At this time of year—and anytime you expect mosquitoes to be buzzing around—you may want to wear protective clothing, such as long sleeves, long pants, and socks. Loose-fitting, light-colored clothing is best. Spray clothing with insect repellent. Remember to follow the instructions on the repellent and to take extra care with children.

CHIGGERS

Chiggers are parasitic mite larvae found on tall grass or other vegetation. They wait for passing hosts, attach themselves to a skin pore or hair follicle, and inject a digestive enzyme that ruptures the cells, causing red, itchy bumps that last for several days. Chiggers are too small to be seen with the naked eye. They are most commonly found in damp areas with a lot of vegetation, and they prefer to attach to skin under tight clothing, such as socks and underwear, or on concealed areas of the body, such as the groin and the armpits. One way to decrease the chance of chigger bites is to wear loose clothing when you're in the woods or other infested areas. You should also take a shower as soon as you get home from an outdoor expedition, to remove any chiggers before they attach to your skin. Keep the irritated area clean, and refrain from scratching. To relieve itching, use a salve or cream that contains antihistamines (Caladryl or hydrocortisone salves are the most common). These will also help to prevent infection. If the welts continue to irritate you for more than a couple of weeks, they might be infected, and you should see a doctor.

EMERALD ASH BORER

This is a warning for anyone planning to build a campfire along the way or on an overnight Ice Age Trail hike, perhaps. The emerald ash borer (*Agrilus planipennis*) is an exotic insect, native to Asia, that currently threatens ash trees in the Great Lakes region. The pest can be spread inadvertently in infested firewood, and most parks have strict rules about what wood you can bring into the park. By following some simple rules, you can help prevent the spread of these destructive insects. Purchase aged firewood near your campsite location; don't bring it from home. Many parks offer firewood at reasonable prices, and it is often available from private sellers just outside the parks. Firewood purchased at or near your destination should be used during your camping trip; don't take any to another destination. Buy wood that has no bark or loose bark (a sign the wood is very dry). This will reduce the chances of infestation while also making your fire easier to start.

SNAKES

Generally speaking, snakes are not a concern in Wisconsin. There are 21 species, but only two are venomous—the Eastern massasauga rattlesnake and the timber rattlesnake—and these are protected as endangered species. You are most likely to see small varieties of garter

PHOTO: Jane Huber

snakes. Although the chances of being bitten by a snake on one of the hikes in this book are practically nil, take proper caution. If you see a snake with a rattle, give it a wide berth.

POISON IVY/POISON OAK/POISON SUMAC

Recognizing poison ivy, oak, and sumac and avoiding contact with them is the most effective way to prevent the painful, itchy rashes associated with these plants. In southern Wisconsin, poison ivy ranges from a thick, tree-hugging vine to a shaded groundcover, three leaflets to a leaf; poison oak occurs as either a vine or a shrub, with three leaflets as well; and poison sumac flourishes in swampland, each leaf containing 7–13 leaflets. Urushiol, the oil in the sap of these plants, is responsible for the rash. Usually within 12–14 hours of exposure (but sometimes much later), raised lines and/or blisters will appear, accompanied by a terrible itch. Refrain from scratching because bacteria under fingernails can cause infection and you will spread the rash to other parts of your body. Wash and dry the rash thoroughly, applying a calamine lotion or other product to help dry the rash. If

PHOTO: Jane Huber

itching or blistering is severe, seek medical attention. Remember that oil-contaminated clothes, pets, or hiking gear can easily cause an irritating rash on you or someone else, so wash not only any exposed parts of your body but also clothes, gear, and pets.

WILD PARSNIP

Wild parsnip, a member of the carrot family, has a long, thick taproot and commonly grows in sunny areas in fields and along roadsides. When conditions are right—usually in the plant's second summer—it sends up a single flower stalk 2–4 feet tall with hundreds of yellow flowers in flat-topped, umbrellalike clusters.

Wild parsnip can cause phytophotodermatitis when the chemicals in the juices of the leaves, stems, and fruits react with ultraviolet light, causing burns to exposed skin. Once absorbed into the skin, the chemicals can be energized by ultraviolet light—even on a cloudy day—causing a burn similar to sunburn in appearance. The skin will redden within 24 to 48 hours and may be accompanied by blisters. A dark red or brown discoloration may also occur and can last as long as two years. Parsnip burns appear as streaks and long spots where a juicy leaf or stem dragged across the skin before exposure to the sun. The burning sensation lasts a day or two. Protective clothing and avoidance are your best protection.

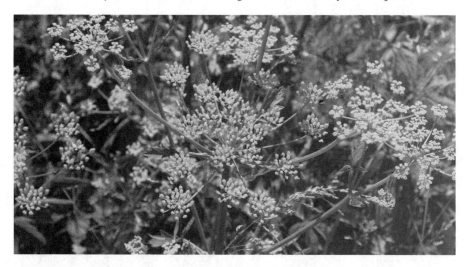

Ice Age Trail Thru-hiking and Dispersed Camping

The portions of the Ice Age Trail in this book are written to stand alone; some segments are out-and-back hikes, while others have been fashioned into loops or lollipops using spur trails or streets to get back to the trailhead. But some hikers may want to thru-hike, or tackle a major section of trail in one direction. The Devil's Lake Segment is an 18-mile example, but, starting from the Brooklyn Wildlife Segment, one can hike all the way to Madison. Indeed, some hikers have tackled the 600-plus miles of finished trail of the projected 1,000 miles planned. To make that possible, the Ice Age Trail Alliance has Dispersed Camping Areas in key locations throughout the trail. Several of them appear in segments within this book. Camping is almost always rustic, with no facilities whatsoever. The rules are simple: Camp within sight of the DCA sign, pack out what you pack in, and wash more than 200 feet from any water source. Camping does not require a permit but is allowed only for thru-hikers and is limited to one night. Human waste should be buried in a 6-inch-deep "cat hole." Campfires are generally not allowed, though you may use a camping stove.

State Natural Areas

Some hikes or portions of them may pass through some of Wisconsin's designated State Natural Areas (SNAs), which are under the jurisdiction of the Department of Natural Resources. These are protected lands offering a view of what Wisconsin looked like before the advent of European settlement and agriculture. Flora and fauna, often rare or threatened species, and terrain have either been preserved or restored to give us a chance to see the state in its original beauty. More than 660 of these areas have received the designation, and as such they have very specific rules for visitors that override rules of adjoining or surrounding parks:

> ➤ SNAs are open 24 hours per day, year-round, unless located within a park with designated hours.

> ➤ Removal of plants and seeds is *prohibited,* with the exception of edibles—wild berries, mushrooms, nuts, herbs, etc.—which can be collected for *personal consumption* only.

> ➤ Removal of any rocks, minerals, trees, or even deadfall/firewood is not permitted.

> ➤ Pets are generally allowed (except within Parfrey's Glen SNA) but on a leash only.

> ➤ All vehicles, including bicycles, are prohibited within the SNA.

> ➤ Except when otherwise indicated, camping and campfires are prohibited.

> ➤ Geocaching is only allowed if the cache is "virtual."

> ➤ Rock climbing is not permitted.

Tips for Enjoying Your Hike

Consider a couple of tips that will make your hike enjoyable and more rewarding:

> ➤ Take your time along the trails. Pace yourself for the longer hikes. The forests, fields, and wetlands of southern Wisconsin are filled with wonders both big and small. Don't rush past a tiny salamander to get to that overlook. Stop and smell the wildflowers. Peer into a clear stream for trout. Don't miss the trees for the forest. Shorter hikes allow you to stop and linger more than long hikes. Something about staring at the front end of a 10-mile trek naturally pushes

you to speed up. That said, take close notice of the elevation maps that accompany each hike. If you see many ups and downs over large altitude changes, you'll obviously need more time. Inevitably, you'll finish some of the hikes long before or after what is suggested. Nevertheless, leave yourself plenty of time for those moments when you simply feel like stopping and taking it all in.

➢ We can't always schedule our free time when we want, but try to hike during the week and avoid the traditional holidays, if possible. Trails that are packed in the summer are often clear during the colder months. If you are hiking on a busy day, go early in the morning; it'll enhance your chances of seeing wildlife. The trails really clear out during rainy times; however, don't hike during a thunderstorm.

➢ Participate in some online wildlife observation counts. Cornell Lab of Ornithology operates **ebird.org,** where you can log in for free and submit bird lists from your hikes or find out what's being seen at some of the area's birding hot spots. A similar count is being done for butterflies at **wisconsinbutterflies.org/butterfly/sightings.**

Trail Etiquette

Whether you're on a city, county, state, or national park trail, always remember that great care and resources (from nature, as well as from your tax dollars) have gone into creating these trails. Treat the trail, wildlife, and fellow hikers with respect.

➢ Hike on open trails only. Respect trail and road closures (ask if not sure), avoid possible trespassing on private land, and obtain all permits and authorization as required. Also, leave gates as you found them or as marked.

➢ Leave only footprints. Be sensitive to the ground beneath you. This also means staying on the existing trail and not blazing any new trails. Be sure to pack out what you pack in. No one likes to see the trash someone else has left behind.

➢ Never spook animals. An unannounced approach, a sudden movement, or a loud noise startles most animals. A surprised animal can be dangerous to you, to others, and to itself. Give them plenty of space.

➢ Plan ahead. Know your equipment, your ability, and the area in which you are hiking—and prepare accordingly. Be self-sufficient at all times; carry necessary supplies for changes in weather or other conditions. A well-executed trip is satisfying to you and to others.

➢ Be courteous to other hikers, bikers, equestrians, and others you encounter on the trails. Greet riders on horseback, rather than slipping deep into the woods to let them pass; this may spook a horse.

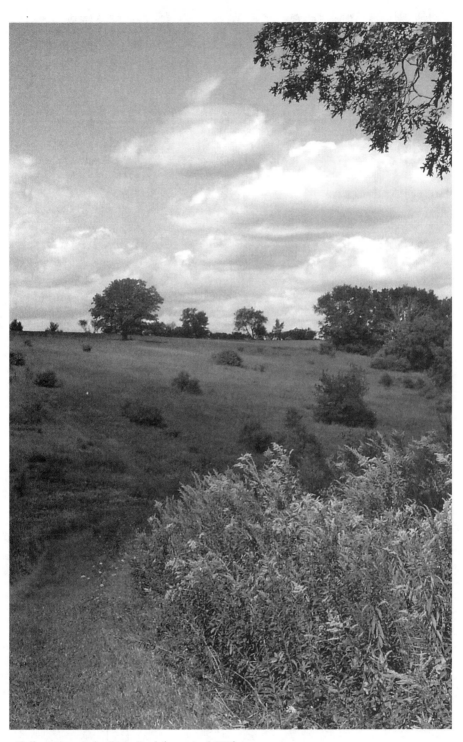

Yellowstone Lake State Park (see page 237)

Madison Metro

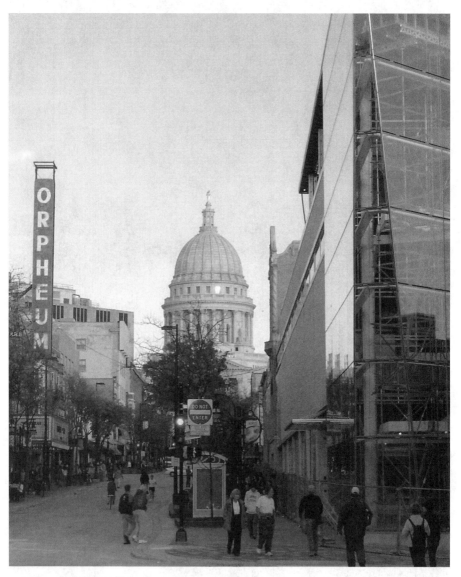

Madison Capitol and Downtown (see page 59)

Madison Metro (Hikes 1–18)

1 Arboretum: Greene Prairie

The trail through Evjue Pine Forest

In Brief

Hike this southernmost portion of the Arboretum and explore oak savanna, pine forest, and one of the finest prairie restorations there is to see.

Description

The centerpiece of this portion of the 1,260-acre University of Wisconsin–Madison Arboretum is Greene Prairie, named for Henry Greene, a UW botanist who, during the 1940s and 1950s, did almost all of the restoration himself, returning what was once farm-land to its original role in the landscape. But the towering pines and oak savanna are no less impressive, and this hike offers a nice mix of all of them.

Take a map from the wooden box at the gate in the parking lot, and then take the packed dirt trail to the left straight into the trees. This first segment takes you through Evjue Pine Forest, parallel to the Beltline Highway, down a lane carpeted with pine nee-dles. The hum of tires will annoy some hikers, but the pine forest has a pleasant airi-ness to it and should not be missed. The rest of this hike is plotted to avoid the nearby urban world.

LENGTH & CONFIGURATION:
2.6-mile loop

DIFFICULTY: Easy, some moderate

SCENERY: Mixed woods, prairie

EXPOSURE: Partly shaded, partly sun

TRAFFIC: Light

TRAIL SURFACE: Packed dirt, crushed stone, exposed rocks and roots, a few narrow boardwalks, potential wet areas

HIKING TIME: 1 hour

DRIVING DISTANCE: At the southeast corner of the intersection of Seminole Highway and the Beltline (US 12/18)

ACCESS: Trails are open 7 a.m.–10 p.m., and parking is from sunrise to sunset.

MAPS: USGS *Madison West;* maps in wooden box at the parking lot or at the visitor center across the highway

WHEELCHAIR ACCESSIBILITY: None

FACILITIES: None

CONTACT: uwarboretum.org, 608-263-7888

COMMENTS: No pets allowed. Check park schedule for free guided tours on weekends. This portion of the park has many trail combinations. Plus, the Arboretum section on the north side of the lake and the central section of the park are listed herein as separate hikes (Arboretum: Wingra Marsh and Arboretum: Wingra Woods).

At 200 feet, you will pass the T2 trail marker, and another 450 feet later, the T3 juncture. Both of these trails break to the right, heading deeper into the pines. Continue straight along here until you arrive at a clearing and trail junction T5, a total of a quarter mile from the trail entrance. Straight across is the trail that will take you about 600 feet to T6 and T7 and a trail that goes left under the Beltline Highway through a tunnel. This is a good way to connect with other great hikes in the Arboretum, in particular Arboretum: Wingra Woods (page 26), and the visitor center, which is found in the central portion of the Arboretum.

By going right (south) at T5, you start to distance yourself from the traffic and avoid the trail along the edge of the Arboretum, which borders a residential neighborhood. Continue through mixed forest; on your right, the pines will eventually give way to oak and other deciduous trees after about 400 feet.

The trail here is a dirt access road. Another 700 feet brings you to the U4 juncture on your right and its trail all the way back to T3. To the left (east) is a trail back to that perimeter path and back to the highway underpass tunnel. Continue straight and you will arrive at a crossroads outside the tree cover 300 feet later at U3. Go left on the crushed stone path and pass scattered trees in savanna as you cross West Grady Knoll. Three hundred feet on, there is a fork in the road. Take the trail that branches to the right at Y1, and to your right you will see prairie grass.

Less than 200 feet in, turn right at the Y2 juncture and, just beyond that at Y3, go right again. The two trails after Y3 are hiking only (no skiing) and run parallel to where they connect a short distance later at Y4. These footpaths are just wide enough for your feet and run through the tall grass and fragile vegetation. You are at the very center of the park, and this little patch of sunlight is a great place to find pasqueflowers and bird's-foot violets in the spring. No matter how tempting, do not pick the flowers.

At the southern end of this segment at Z1, the path rejoins the ski trail. Turn right here (passing what will be your return trail just a few steps from where you just joined this path) and follow the gently curving trail through the southern edge of Grady Oak Savanna. At the next juncture 500 feet later, pass the trail at Z2, which connects back up the hill to Y2 where you left it. Continue straight across, pass a connecting trail into the prairie at Z3, and hike 0.2 mile along the bottom of the slope of the savanna and just south of East Knoll, bringing you to the Z4 juncture. Go right and you will come to a path just 200 feet farther on that enters into the heart of Greene Prairie. (A spur trail on the left leads into nearby Knollwood Conservation Park.)

Held up as one of the finest examples of prairie restoration in the world, the prairie receives periodic controlled burns in spring, which park administrators hope will protect that restoration. Urban development to the south has affected water runoff, and, unfortunately, the park is now faced with losing the prairie to reed canary grass, an invasive species. This is best to visit in spring, when a wide variety of wildflowers bloom. But also during this time and in rainy periods, the trail can get soggy here and you might get your feet wet.

The trail does a 0.4-mile half loop through this southeastern corner of the park. When you come to Z6 at 0.3 mile, take the two-plank boardwalk to your left. This takes you back across the prairie and leaves you at the packed-earth trail that re-enters the oak savanna through pussy willows. Go left here at Z1. To your left are quaking aspens. You pass through 750 feet of younger trees before arriving at X3, heading left, and crossing 500 feet of the northernmost finger of Greene Prairie to arrive at the X5 juncture. If you continue straight, you can hike all the way to the southernmost edge of the park, follow the trail west around Southwest Grady Oak Savanna, and then head north through the forest along Seminole Highway. This adds only about a quarter mile to the hike, but this area is also prone to sogginess. Going right takes you through the woods on a very rudimentary and sometimes muddy trail. Make no mistake: This is not oak savanna but mixed forest.

When you arrive at X6, go right and follow the trail through the woods all the way back to the trailhead and parking lot. Along the way, you will pass the V1 and X1 trail outlets and finally the U1 outlet just 500 feet from the end.

Nearby Activities

Just 1 mile south of here on the right on Seminole Highway is a nicely paved bike trail at Dunn's Marsh. Continue south to the next traffic light intersection to find McKee Road/County Road PD.

GPS COORDINATES AND DIRECTIONS
N43° 02' 2.99" W89° 26' 36.24"

Follow the Beltline (US 12/18) west to the Seminole Highway exit. Go left on the overpass and through the four-way stop on the other side. The small gravel parking lot is immediately on your left at the corner. There is no exit from the Beltline here if you are going east. In this case, take the Todd Drive exit and take your first right to go back the opposite direction to the same Seminole Highway four-way stop. Turn left and immediately left again into the lot at the corner.

2 Arboretum: Wingra Marsh

A spring creek on the north side of Lake Wingra

In Brief

Step from the sidewalk in a popular west side neighborhood onto a trail through the marsh and forest along Lake Wingra's northwest shore.

Description

The Arboretum is made up of 1,200 acres of preserved land and, combined with Vilas Park, almost completely encompasses Lake Wingra. It all looks very pristine and natural, so it is hard to believe that this was all once farmland. Much of the land was purchased during the Great Depression, and, with the help of Civilian Conservation Corps workers and ecologists such as Aldo Leopold, it was set on the path to become the astounding restoration of prairie, forests, and wetlands that we see today. This segment that curls around the northwestern shore of the lake is an easily accessible hike that never strays far from a busy street and yet offers as much natural beauty as the heart of the park.

The hike begins with a spring bubbling up from under a sandstone wall off Nakoma Road. There are a couple of benches along a mowed area right next to the parking lot where you can sit and watch waterfowl. The trail starts from the lot on a multiuse asphalt path shared by bicyclists, but, only 250 feet in, a narrow footpath departs to the right into

LENGTH & CONFIGURATION: 1.6-mile out-and-back	**ACCESS:** Trails are open 7 a.m.–10 p.m., and parking is sunrise–sunset.
DIFFICULTY: Easy	**MAPS:** USGS *Madison West;* park maps inside wooden boxes at trail entrances
SCENERY: Mixed forest, marsh	
EXPOSURE: Mostly shaded	**WHEELCHAIR ACCESSIBILITY:** None
TRAFFIC: Moderate	**FACILITIES:** Restrooms at boat livery in Wingra Park
TRAIL SURFACE: Mostly wood chip and packed dirt, some boardwalk and asphalt	**CONTACT:** uwarboretum.org
HIKING TIME: 45 minutes	**COMMENTS:** Public tours and other programs take place on most weekends at the Arboretum. Contact the visitor center at 608-263-7888. Pets are prohibited.
DRIVING DISTANCE: 1.7 miles west of Monroe and Regent Streets	

the forest. (The multiuse trail runs along the edge of the park all the way to a connection with Arbor Drive.) The underbrush is thick here, but 200 feet in, you arrive at the edge of the Marion Dunn Marsh and follow along the top of the earthen dike.

Look for turtles perched on rocks along the shore and expect a chorus of frogs. Another 200 feet farther, the land opens to Marion Dunn Prairie with a few scattered trees, some of them dead and barren, perfect for perching hawks and crows.

You can now see Lake Wingra to the south through the trees. The trail curls around this pocket of marsh and comes close to a busy three-way intersection on Monroe and Glenway Streets, where there is another entry point to the trail at marker Q1. There, in a wooden box, you will also find trail maps for the entire Arboretum. It is also possible to park your car across the street and down one of the residential side streets.

Continue through the tall grass another 100 feet and you are in the shade of the trees once again. You come to trail marker Q5, where another spur trail to the left connects to Monroe Street. Wildflowers are abundant here in the spring, especially bird's-foot violets.

The trail splits here at marker R2. Going straight bypasses a 350-foot loop to the marsh. Take the two-plank boardwalk to the right and follow it to the edge of the water, which is an inlet almost cut off from the rest of the lake. This is Ho Nee Um Pond and is almost guaranteed to have a few Canada geese or mallards lurking about. Still water stretches out to a long, narrow spit of land with the last line of trees between the marsh and the open lake. There are a lot of dead trees in this area. Keep an eye out for flickers and woodpeckers.

The loop passes the edge of the stagnant water and soon returns to the main trail at marker R3. Head right, and 100 feet later cross a spring. You can see the water bubbling up through the sand at the bottom. Water bugs play across the surface in the summer, and in the winter it is often still green with moss back here.

Arboretum: Wingra Marsh

Another 100 feet later, the trail crosses another spring large enough to become a creek. The boardwalk comes only to the edge of the water, and you must cross 10 feet on stepping-stones. Then the boardwalk resumes but ends just 50 feet beyond. On your left is a trail that takes you less than 50 feet to a council ring, and beyond that to a parking lot off Arbor Drive. But, continuing on the main trail here, the park opens to an area of regularly maintained grass. Stay right and look for the concrete culvert that crosses the trail. To your right is the edge of the open water again, with waterfowl hiding out and an abundance of dragonflies.

The footpath trail resumes nearby and passes beneath a few maples as it follows Arbor Drive. You cross a runoff channel 200 feet farther on and walk along the edge of Ho Nee Um Pond. Keep going another 200 feet and go right at the fork in the trail, staying inside the park. One hundred feet farther, the trail forks again. The path to the left is your return trail. Go right and follow the pond's edge 250 feet out to the point. A handful of spurs make the few steps to the water.

As the shoreline forces the trail to curve left, enter a patch of cedars, pass a small dock out into Lake Wingra on your right, and, only 200 feet later, arrive at the far end of the trail and another entry point from Wingra Park. You will pass a storage shed on your left before exiting the woods behind the boat livery at Wingra Park. The northbound forest trail has been closed, so you need to exit the woods and follow along the edge of the parking lot, heading north to pick up the trail as it re-enters the trees near the entrance to the lot at Arbor Drive and Knickerbocker Street. This is trail point R6.

Watch the trail for deer prints; it's not unheard of for them to venture this far into the city. This trail brings you back to the fork where you went right at the pond's edge. Here you can follow the trail in reverse to return to the parking lot, exit to the street to take the sidewalk back, or go a block north to Monroe Street to restaurants and shops. The multiuse trail is another return-trip option.

Nearby Activities

Monroe Street neighborhood has several nice restaurants, and a Madison classic, Michael's Frozen Custard, is at the heart of it at 2531 Monroe St. (608-231-3500). You can rent canoes at Wingra Boats (608-233-5332 or **wingraboats.com**), located in Wingra Park at the easternmost point of this trail.,

---

GPS COORDINATES AND DIRECTIONS
N43° 03' 1.50" W89° 26' 12.21"

Follow Monroe Street 1.7 miles west from where it intersects Regent Street downtown to where it splits into Odana Road and Nakoma Road. Take the curve left to Nakoma, and just half a block farther, you will find the parking lot on your left. The trail begins on the asphalt bike path from the parking lot.

3 Arboretum: Wingra Woods

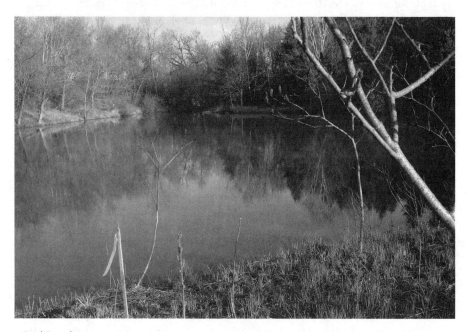

Teal Pond

In Brief

Find the springs that feed Lake Wingra, visit the gardens, and explore the 1,200 acres of forest and prairie at the heart of the city.

Description

The University of Wisconsin's Arboretum is not your standard labeled garden. With more than 1,200 acres of restored wetlands, prairies, savannas, and woods, it is a remarkable ecological preserve in the heart of a city. Most of this land was purchased in the Great Depression, and the Civilian Conservation Corps did much of the initial work to set it up. Outside of Longenecker Gardens—which is a more traditional arboretum gathering more than 100 species of Wisconsin woody plants in 50 acres—the preserve looks simply like undeveloped landscape and gives little indication of the ongoing preservation and reclamation efforts.

The trailhead is at the west end of the parking lot opposite the wooden sign and map box, which is at the head of another cutoff trail. Across the road to the south is the entrance to Longenecker Gardens, where you'll find a bike rack and map box.

LENGTH & CONFIGURATION:
2.4-mile loop

DIFFICULTY: Easy to moderate

SCENERY: Mixed woods, natural springs, ponds, American Indian effigy mounds

EXPOSURE: Mostly shaded

TRAFFIC: Moderate to light

TRAIL SURFACE: Packed dirt, a few narrow boardwalks, exposed rocks and roots

HIKING TIME: 1 hour

DRIVING DISTANCE: 2.8 miles from the intersection of Fish Hatchery Road and Park Street

ACCESS: Trails are open 7 a.m.–10 p.m., and parking is sunrise–sunset.

MAPS: USGS *Madison West;* maps in the wooden boxes at trailheads

WHEELCHAIR ACCESSIBILITY: None

FACILITIES: Restrooms at the nearby visitor center

CONTACT: uwarboretum.org

COMMENTS: Pets are prohibited. This central portion of the park has a wide variety of trail combinations. Plus, the Arboretum section on the north side of the lake and the southern section of the park are listed herein as separate hikes (Arboretum: Greene Prairie and Arboretum: Wingra Marsh).

The trail passes over exposed rocks and tree roots or under leaves, skirting along the park road 700 feet before turning down through oak savanna with Overlook Prairie to your left. If you go left at trail marker M1, the path takes you along the prairie 700 feet and then back onto the Arboretum Drive. Go right here, as the trail curves down the hill at a gentle grade as it gets closer to the lake. This is also a cross-country ski trail; if you are hiking this in winter (which is a great hike), skiers have the right-of-way.

Expect a lot of fallen wood as you hike 0.2 mile to the lowest point of the trail. To the left are the springs that feed Lake Wingra. Also on your left is a two-plank boardwalk. Follow this into the marshy area to see the water up close. This 400-foot loop comes back to the trail you just left only 50 feet down the trail at M7.

Just beyond this is a stone platform with a railing and a bench. You can almost see the lake through the brush. It remains green here, just inside the water, even in winter. To the right, a cutoff trail leads back to the parking lot with a moderate grade. That trail cuts through some American Indian effigy mounds.

Continue along the marsh's edge another 700 feet and find another large spring on your left. You encounter more rocks on the trail here and other smaller springs to the left before you head into some pines. At junction K4, go right. Going straight will take you out to Arboretum Drive. Uphill from K4 on a mild grade, cross gentle hills for 350 feet, and at the top find a bench at the K2 junction. To your right, another trail cuts back to the parking lot, but stay the course to arrive at Arboretum Drive just another 700 feet across level terrain. At the gate here is a good place to lock up a bike if you want to jump on the trail in the middle. A crosswalk and a narrow twisting gate keep out dogs and bikes. There is also another map box here.

Now you are entering Gallistel Woods. Four hundred feet from the road at the first junction (G5), go left, walk another 100 feet to another juncture (G4), and again go left to

Arboretum: Wingra Woods

Lost City Forest

enter the Lost City Forest. In 1916, this was an ill-chosen development project, but nature had its way: The soggy substrata simply swallowed up most of what was laid down on it, and so there are woods where there would have been suburbs. Go 130 feet past the G4 junction and cross a creek that drains all the way to the lake. This is the least developed section of the trail, and though easy to follow, it can get muddy, and the boardwalk does not go the entire length of the segment. Still, this is nice and secluded, and you can observe a lot of wildlife through here. The trail heads south nearly 0.4 mile until it reaches junction L4, a four-way intersection, at a crushed-stone access lane.

Go straight across into a section of conifers and take the hiking-only trail. Meander 400 feet through the woods to rejoin the ski trail you just crossed. This brings you to L3 where you head south (left), though another trail heads west from here. About 300 feet past here, you can see an industrial park through the trees to your left, and to the right you find the creatively named Pond Two (the second Teal Pond). Pass the trail to your right at L2 and continue past the pond's edge to L1 before turning right across a concrete runoff channel to circle the pond. The trail is well shaded here along the pond's south shore, and a bench 130 feet in offers a nice respite. At the next trail juncture, the trail offers a stroll through the Leopold Pines along the highway to the left. This hike, however, continues to the right passing Pond Two on your right and then Teal Pond Wetlands. At the next juncture, turn right across the north side of the wetlands, staying right again at the F1 juncture. Expect abundant birds in here. At juncture F2, go left. Immediately on your right at F3 is a short spur trail east to a platform overlooking Teal Pond.

Continue another 300 feet to the F4 juncture, where a path to the left also sends you via Juniper Knoll to Curtis Prairie and Leopold Pines. There is much to see out in that direction, but the path chosen here keeps you from the noise of the Beltline Highway, which passes just south of this section of the Arboretum. At its southwesternmost point, there is a tunnel under the highway to reach the southern portion of the park and the Arboretum: Green Prairie hike (page 18).

Continue another 250 feet; then turn right at F6. Walk 300 feet to come upon Gallistel Shelter House for skiers to the left. To the right is a spur trail that takes you to a nice board-walk that ends with a viewing platform. This area is open to the sun and full of cattails, frogs, and marsh birds. The boardwalk has a couple of observation benches along the way.

Return to the Gallistel Shelter and head right 250 feet where the trail starts to get a little steeper. Go left at juncture G1, which begins the steepest portion of the trail. It's about a 500-foot moderate-grade climb, and halfway up is a bench if you need a rest or want to take in a patch of wildflowers in the spring.

On your right at the G6 juncture is an American Indian mound. Take the trail left, and 400 feet later exit the woods. Pass through the gardens along the fence line to the right to find the exit, but this is a nice place to linger, especially in April and early May when all the trees are in bloom.

Nearby Activities

The Arboretum offers public tours, scheduled guided hikes, and other activities on most weekends and in most weather. Go to **uwarboretum.org,** call 608-263-7888, or check the seasonal map/brochures found in wooden boxes at park entrances to find out the schedule. The Vilas Zoo is located just across Lake Wingra in Vilas Park. Arboretum Drive will take you there along the southern shore of Lake Wingra and is popular with runners, bikers, and walkers.

GPS COORDINATES AND DIRECTIONS
N43° 02' 43.88" W89° 25' 40.36"

Go south 0.5 mile on Fish Hatchery Road from where it begins at its intersection with Park Street. At the first traffic light, go right on Wingra Road 0.5 mile and turn left on Arboretum Drive. Follow this 1.8 miles along the lake and through the woods until you find the parking lot on your right across from Longenecker Gardens.

4 Capital City State Trail: E-Way Segment

The paved trail passes through fields of wildflowers.

In Brief

This popular multiuse trail on smooth asphalt takes you from the east side to the west side of Madison via wetlands, prairie, and a long greenway tucked into a residential area.

Description

From the entrance of Lake Farm County Park, cross Lake Farm Road and start down the asphalt Capital City State Trail. The trail also goes north from here on the east side of the road, continuing all the way up along Lake Monona and eventually to the east side of Madison.

The trail starts out through prairie. At 0.3 mile, you pass a park bench and some picnic tables just after that as the trail winds 0.2 mile through oak forest. Beyond that, the prairie of the Lewis Nine Springs E-Way is to your right and chock-full of wildflowers, including bergamot, coneflowers, Queen Anne's lace, and black-eyed Susans. A spur trail connects through the prairie to the Lewis Nine Springs E-Way trail, and this portion of the Capital City Trail is currently the return path for that hike, which begins just north of here. You might see deer and wild turkeys through these fields.

Agricultural fields begin on your left 0.3 mile from the forest, and you really seem far from the city. Continue 0.4 mile and pick up a bit of oak savanna on your left just before

LENGTH & CONFIGURATION: 8-mile point-to-point or 16-mile out-and-back	**ACCESS:** Year-round
	MAPS: USGS *Madison West* and *Madison East;* map boards at trailheads
DIFFICULTY: Easy	
SCENERY: Prairie, mixed forest, marsh	**WHEELCHAIR ACCESSIBILITY:** Yes
EXPOSURE: Mostly sun	**FACILITIES:** None on trail; restrooms and water at Lake Farm County Park near trailhead and Nevin Fish Hatchery, just off the trail on Fish Hatchery Road
TRAFFIC: Moderate	
TRAIL SURFACE: Asphalt	
HIKING TIME: 3–3.5 hours	**CONTACT:** dnr.wi.gov/topic/parks/name/capcity, 608-224-3730
DRIVING DISTANCE: 1.5 miles south of the Beltline Highway US 12/18 and South Towne Drive	**COMMENTS:** Bicyclists must pay a state trail fee ($4 daily, $20 annual). Leashed dogs allowed.

you come to the corner of Larsen Road and East Clayton Road. To your right, an access road leads to a pump station behind a metal gate. Currently, this is officially off-limits. In the future, there are hopes to get the right-of-way and use this corridor as a return trail for the Lewis Nine Springs E-Way trail.

The trail continues along Clayton Road with cropland to your right. At 0.3 mile the path climbs moderately as you approach a curve to the right that takes the path around the right side of a small ridge that separates it from the road for a short stretch. At the top of the hill, a trail goes to the right along a row of trees. This is where the Lewis Nine Springs E-Way trail first joins this trail on its return in the opposite direction. There is a bench at the top of the hill overlooking the fields to the right.

From the bench, it's another 0.3 mile to County Road MM, with the trail following close to the edge of Clayton Road. At the next corner, cross MM and go right along the sidewalk, immediately crossing McCoy Road. Go left on the other side and cross the on-ramp to US 14, go under the overpass, and cross the ramp on the other side. The trail continues from here along McCoy Road.

The next 0.7 mile takes you along marshland to the right with a line of cottonwoods granting a bit of shade at times, but the trail is mostly exposed. Wildflowers line the trail. At 0.5 mile, cross railroad tracks before reaching Syene Road 0.2 mile later.

Go straight across to a parking area on the right. The next 0.6 mile crosses through a bit of prairie and brush before heading into oak forest and public hunting grounds. There is no shade, however. Another 0.2 mile later, long-needle pines close in around the trail. You'll pass a bench just before the trail curves right with thick underbrush on either side. This is the most remote point on the trail.

From the bench at 0.2 mile, find a spur trail that rides parallel, an older version of the current trail. This loops off left through some prairie and crosses a small bridge before it rejoins the main trail again 800 feet farther on. Just past this, the trail enters woods for 0.1 mile, and then the path is open to the sky for the next 0.4 mile as it passes behind a school

Capital City State Trail: E-Way Segment

and climbs a hill up to Gunflint Trail. Follow this right to Glacier Valley Road. Take this to the right 0.3 mile through residences until it meets Fish Hatchery Road. To your right is the Nevin Fish Hatchery, which offers tours, restrooms, water, and park information during business hours. Take the sidewalk to the left 0.1 mile to head up a loop for the pedestrian/bike bridge across Fish Hatchery Road at the traffic light at McKee Road.

The trail resumes on the other side, going along the top of a ridge and then bearing right away from the intersection and the busy roads as it descends into a corridor of forest with a certain secret-garden quality to it.

Cross two bridges in the first 0.3 mile, and then reach a short tunnel under Longford Terrace another 0.3 mile after that. It is quiet back here, but beware of bikers flying past around tight turns. A small creek trickles through around large rocks to your right, and the trail is mostly shaded by oaks.

Another 0.4 mile takes you across Edenberry Street through exposed terrain and finally into a mowed park area. This 0.3-mile stretch winds through the park slightly uphill and takes you to a wooded segment—the last 0.4 mile out to Seminole Highway, with condos to the right just outside the trees.

After crossing the busy street, the trail curves 0.3 mile through wildflowers, with a drainage area/wetlands to the right, where you might see a lot of birds, especially during migration periods. Prairie is to your left, as is a spur trail to the parking area for Dunn Marsh. This is another good entry point to the trail.

Enter a wooded area after this and continue 0.4 mile until you come to a trail juncture. Cross the Cannonball Path as you pass under a bridge, which is the overpass for the Badger State Trail. Stay on the Capital City Trail; just past here, an asphalt trail goes right. This is the Southwest Path, which leads all the way downtown to Camp Randall Stadium and connects with the Badger State Trail above you, just a short walk from where you're standing. Stay straight here; the last 0.3 mile of the trail curves left past a pond on the right, then a playground, and finally another pond on the left before curling uphill to the end of the trail. There are no facilities there but a map board.

Nearby Activities

Lake Farm County Park at the head of the trail has some short trails in and around the marsh, and the Lussier Family Heritage Center provides information about the history of the area.

GPS COORDINATES AND DIRECTIONS
N43° 01' 38.02" W89° 20' 43.10"

From the Beltline Highway (US 12/18), go south 0.8 mile on South Towne Drive (which becomes Raywood Road) to Moorland Road. Go left and drive 0.7 mile, even as the road bends right and becomes Lake Farm Road. This will bring you to the parking lot for Lake Farm Park/Centennial Springs State Park on your left and the trailhead on your right, directly across from the park entrance.

5 Cherokee Marsh North

This observation platform is along the boardwalk trail where you are likely to spot, or at least hear, sandhill cranes.

In Brief

Find many species of birds along trails through prairie and boardwalks through the wetlands at this rich marsh along the Yahara River just north of Lake Mendota.

Description

Madison's famous chain of four lakes is the beneficiary of the Upper Yahara River, which, together with the Cherokee Marsh, drains the lands north of Lake Mendota. At 3,200 acres, the marsh is the largest wetland in Dane County.

Ten thousand years ago, the retreating glaciers created a lake here, covering much more territory than the present-day Mendota. The fine sediments left behind did not promote drainage, so the soil above them remained saturated, forming wetlands. With wetlands comes the partially decayed vegetable matter known as peat, which is up to 10 feet thick in some places.

Nineteenth-century farmers couldn't use this land, so they did all they could to drain it. Perhaps all of the marsh would have been lost had the locals not put in a dam at the outlet of Lake Mendota in 1850, thus backing up water and making the areas we have today impossible to drain.

If it's not one threat, it's another; more than 640 acres of the marsh eroded after that dam went in. The raised lake levels caused the buoyant peat to become floating bogs. Residential development in the 1960s caused a major tract of these bobbing sedge meadows to break free, creating the widened part of the Yahara known as Cherokee Lake. Wetland restoration efforts have gone a long way in returning the marsh to a healthier state,

LENGTH & CONFIGURATION:
2-mile double loop

DIFFICULTY: Easy to moderate

SCENERY: Mixed forest, prairie, and wetlands

EXPOSURE: Mostly sun, with partial shade in the wooded stretch

TRAFFIC: Light

TRAIL SURFACE: Crushed stone, packed dirt, grass, and boardwalks

HIKING TIME: 1 hour

DRIVING DISTANCE: 2 miles north on Sherman Avenue from the Northport Drive intersection

ACCESS: Open 4 a.m.–1 hour after sunset

MAPS: USGS *De Forest;* posted on map board in parking lot

WHEELCHAIR ACCESSIBILITY: Restrooms and some trails

FACILITIES: Restrooms, picnic tables, bike rack, water fountain

CONTACT: cityofmadison.com/parks/cherokeenorth

COMMENTS: No dogs allowed. This is listed as a birding hot spot at Cornell University's **ebird.org.**

and what we have today is a rich environment for a variety of flora and fauna. Additionally, recent burns and tree removal have done an impressive job of reviving oak savanna, which in turn has brought back many species of wildflowers and birds, such as the red-headed woodpecker.

From the north end of the parking lot, go north on crushed rock, crossing an access road before entering the trees. The trail bends to the right, and then a branch heads out into the open on a mowed path. Pass this by and stay left inside the aspens. At the next four-way intersection 300 feet later, go straight across. The path to the left leads to other short trails through the woods and where the long boardwalk used to be. The path to the right is a cutoff that will skip the woods on the hill and the prairie beyond, taking you right back to the marshy area. Stay straight on the crushed-stone access road that slopes down on a couple of boardwalks out to viewing platforms over the marsh and the Yahara River. There was once an extensive boardwalk trail south of here, but, unfortunately, a park manager decided to take it out, citing environmental reasons.

Continue on down the access road, and, 800 feet later, a trail rises up to the right. The access road continues down to the water's edge. The trail rises into the forest at a moderate grade.

Not long after cresting the hill just over 0.2 mile later, you come out of the forest to a bench overlooking a long slope of prairie that extends down to a pond in a small stand of woods. To the right is a cutoff trail that takes you back down and around this hill and directly to the wetlands. Continue straight down the hill, taking the grassy trail to your left. Cross 0.2 mile of open meadow to a clump of trees at the bottom of the slope. Inside is a small pond with a boardwalk and platform that extends into the middle of it. Frogs and dragonflies are active here.

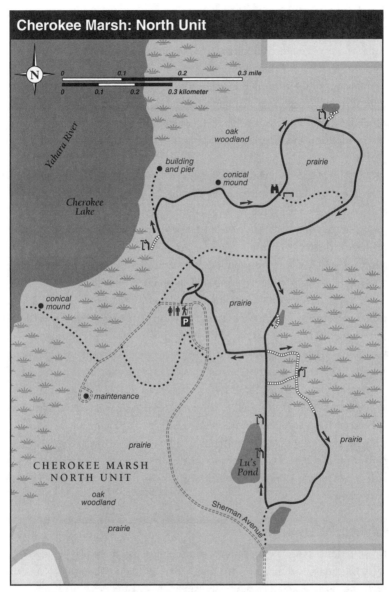

Cherokee Marsh: North Unit

The trail then turns back up the hill another 0.2 mile and comes to the cutoff juncture still within sight of the bench at the top. Pass over the ridge and descend along the edge of the woods where the trail turns back into the shade for 200 feet before coming to a three-way intersection. Go left here, and the trail ventures out toward the marshy areas. Only 0.2 mile later, you hit another juncture. To the right cuts back to the parking lot, but go straight for your return trail. Go left onto the boardwalk, which meanders into the marsh to a raised viewing platform 400 feet in. Listen for sandhill cranes here. The added height of the platform should give you better odds of spotting one and several other species of birds.

Just past the platform, a cutoff trail takes you back out of the marsh, but continue straight for another 400 feet to reach the end of the planks. When the trail leaves the boardwalk, expect to have some tricky going if there has been any amount of rainfall. Waterproof footwear or sandals are your best bet here, though during dry periods, you generally have little to worry about.

Follow the trail in a long loop south that cuts through prairie before returning to less spongy terrain and slightly higher ground at 0.2 mile. At the first juncture, find a trail heading left to the park gates. Continuing, however, go right, heading back north. Along this crushed-rock trail, you come across two viewing platforms leaning toward the marsh to the left. However, they are not raised like the previous one. This return segment of the loop takes you a quarter mile back to the entrance to the boardwalk (you pass the boardwalk cutoff trail first). Turn left here, and go 300 feet to where another exit takes you to the southern end of the parking lot. But stay on the trail and go right across the prairie for another 600 feet, bringing you back to the forest trail near where you started the hike. Head left and go 100 feet, taking another left to exit to the parking lot.

This park is excellent for bird-watching, and you can expect to see plenty of waterfowl, herons, and cranes. In April, you will find many migratory species. Share your observations at Cornell University's **ebird.org,** where you can also see what others are seeing and when.

Nearby Activities

The Madison Mallards are a college-level summer baseball team playing at Warner Park near North Sherman Avenue and Northport Drive. Find out when there's a home game by going to **mallardsbaseball.com** or calling 608-246-4277.

GPS COORDINATES AND DIRECTIONS
N43° 10' 1.51" W89° 21' 53.05"

On the northeast side of Lake Mendota, North Sherman Avenue intersects Northport Drive (WI 113). Follow Sherman Avenue 2 miles north, passing Cherokee Country Club and ending right at the park entrance. Continue to the parking lot to find the trailhead. If the gates are closed, you can park outside them and follow a trail on the right that will take you straight north to the parking lot and trailhead.

6 Cherokee Marsh South

Cherokee Creek joins the Yahara River.

In Brief

Cross open fields and wetlands, and hike up and down small hills in oak forest, as you find viewpoints along this trail through the lower portion of Cherokee Marsh along the Yahara River.

Description

The damming of Lake Mendota kept Cherokee Marsh from being drained for agriculture in the late 19th century, but it wasn't just the pioneers that dealt with land management. Native Americans once set fires to maintain the open fields. The marsh area remains important as it filters out excess fertilizer from upland runoff, helping to keep the lakes cleaner.

The park is the focus of wetland, prairie, and oak savanna restoration projects, and many species of birds, such as the marsh hawk and the short-eared owl, benefit from these efforts. This is the lower portion of the marsh closest to where the Yahara River, which runs through it, empties into Lake Mendota.

If the gates in front of the park entry road are closed, you can still park there and pick up the trail at a point to the left of the gate. The gravel parking lot at the end of the entry road has a small dock on Cherokee Creek that feeds into the Yahara River to the west.

LENGTH & CONFIGURATION: 3-mile out-and-back with interconnected loops	north of Northport Drive (WI 113) and School Road
DIFFICULTY: Easy to moderate	**ACCESS:** 4 a.m.–sunset
SCENERY: Mixed forest, prairie, and wetlands, river views	**MAPS:** USGS *Waunakee*
	WHEELCHAIR ACCESSIBILITY: None
EXPOSURE: Shaded and sunny portions	**FACILITIES:** None
TRAFFIC: Light	**CONTACT:** cityofmadison.com/parks/cherokeesouth
TRAIL SURFACE: Packed dirt, some crushed stone	**COMMENTS:** Bring bug spray. Portions of this trail can be soggy, especially after rain, so plan your footwear accordingly. No dogs allowed.
HIKING TIME: 1.5–2 hours	
DRIVING DISTANCE: 0.75 mile	

Look for the trailhead next to a cottonwood to the left as you enter the lot where you'll find a small sign that says CONSERVATION PARK and a wire across the entry.

Step around or duck under the wire to find the grassy trail splitting left and right. Head left away from the creek. The trail goes up gently; in summer the grass may be higher than your head. As you gain a little altitude on the hill, you get an overview of the cattails to the left across the entry road. To the right, the ridge is still higher than you, so you don't see the river beyond the other side.

At 550 feet from the trailhead, find a wooden post where the trail goes right up the hill or down to the left. You can see water in the distance from here to the right. Go down the path to the left and find a marshy area to the right, where you might come across cranes and herons on their spindly legs searching for a meal. The path follows along the edge of the entry road for another 500 feet until you arrive at a transformer station. Cut stumps are graying in the sun to your right in more soggy terrain. The deadwood makes a nice home for shelf fungi. Beyond this, you enter a maintained area around a brick service building, and the trail seems to disappear. Staying in front of the building, follow a direct line across the lot to arrive at the other side and pick up the cut-grass trail again.

The trail shows some sandy spots, and, in summer, you see many ant mounds along the way. Two hundred feet from the brick building, enter the woods through a stand of cottonwoods and pussy willows. Trail grass can get long here, but it is generally maintained. Here is one of the segments of the trail that affords a bit of shade. The trail can get soggy and even muddy back here. Reach the first trail juncture 400 feet into the trees. The trail to the right goes up the hill through the trees and is a cutoff to the return trail. It is also higher ground if the terrain is soggy elsewhere. But go left at this juncture through a small clearing. The low area to the left shows fallen trees and marsh. At the next intersection, go left as you cross over a ditch full of stagnant water and, needless to say, mosquitoes in season. Go straight across the next juncture, following the trail to the edge of the park, where it turns left. Telephone wires and power lines mark the street to the right,

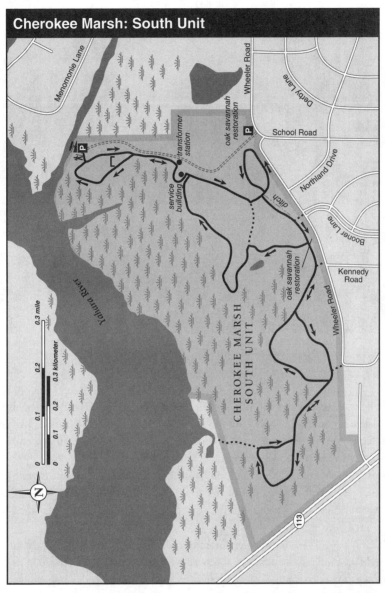

Cherokee Marsh: South Unit

Looking out over wetlands to the Yahara River from a hillock of aspens

and thick brush separates you from a residential neighborhood. Follow along about 500 feet and you'll come to a short trail to the right that leads to the outside parking lot. Instead, continue left here around the loop another 500 feet as the trail descends gently. Go right at the juncture and take an immediate left, entering a wide clearing. The brush and the ditch pass along the left, and, on your right, a gash in the woods is wide open to the sky. Come out of this section of the trail 500 feet later at cedar chips and an oak savanna restoration area. To your left is an exit trail 50 feet to Wheeler Road. Street parking and entry here are also possible.

Halfway across the 600-foot section of oak plantings, pass a wooden post and a trail to the right up a hill into woods. The southernmost section of the trail is a loop from here, and this is your return route. So keep straight along here to the end, where your trail goes right at another juncture; you can also exit to Wheeler Road to the left. The trail is uneven with the natural shape of the ground.

This garden to your left was cleared of box elders in 2007 to make way for some oak saplings. Previously, the taller and faster-growing box elders were edging out the oaks, causing them to grow into the road in search of sunlight. The buckthorn and honeysuckle understory was also cleared. Fifteen oaks have been planted here, and over time it will look less like a garden as the understory overpowers the cedar chips.

Following the trail right away from the road, you immediately pass a big boulder to the right and see dead trees standing out of brush in a marshy area. Lots of cottonwoods

Cattails at the edge of the marsh

stand here as you pass through deeper into marsh 500 feet to the first juncture. Go left; the straight path is your return from the big loop.

Pass through some shrubs and then cross prairie marsh, with grasses undulating in the wind and the occasional mourning doves bursting from hiding as you pass. To the left is the residential street over the tall grasses, and you can hear the highway in the distance.

A trail goes left out to Wheeler Road, and as you continue another 100 feet, you pass a post marking your return trail to the right. Go straight here where the trail shows a bit of crushed rock. The road is firm and crosses through marsh on both sides until you arrive 300 feet later at the edge of more woods. In the wetlands, tall gray trunks stand like columns to the left and redwing blackbirds keep up a constant chatter. This is the closest point to WI 113, and the hum of wheels can distract, yet it is surprising how much animal activity you find here. You are likely to spot deer among the oaks. At the first trail juncture, go left; the right is the return path. The trail takes you on a 0.3-mile loop back to this point, with oak leaves covering tree roots along the path. You may find some unofficial side trails into the underbrush, but stay on the main trail to complete the loop. One exception is about two-thirds of the way around the loop: a spur trail, wide and clear on the left of the next fork, that takes you 400 feet straight to the water's edge for a clearer look. Return to the loop and head back out into the marsh until you come once again to the wooden post.

Go left here, and the trail dips down to its lowest and marshiest point. This whole segment is going to give you soakers in rainy periods, but higher ground comes in 350 feet or so. This affords a view of the water far ahead and the rising opposite bank of the river. But the view is short-lived, because brush envelops you 200 feet farther on and the trail rejoins the return to the oak savanna 600 feet after that. Once you reach the savanna again, go left to that wooden post and break left into the woods. Look for raspberries on the left side of the path here in July. The trail goes uphill on crushed rock. When you crest the small hill, you walk along the top before the path curls left and descends again through the dip between this hill and the next. Just beyond the trees to the left is standing water. At the top of the next hill, the path doubles back. Head down again, then up again, and once again you double back, making a 900-foot S-trail through the oaks.

Exit the woods at a post with a broken piece of chain on the left. The trail goes right and left. Go left into the sun, with trees on your left and grassy fields with milkweed and Indian paintbrush to the right. The path rises sharply and crests the hill, and you are granted a view back across the marshy area toward the highway where you've just been. The curve brings you around the end of this field to head back the other direction, this time with the trees to your left and the grasses to your right. Pass through some oaks and some young aspens to the right. To the left is a narrow stretch of trees that marks the edge of the higher ground and the marsh beyond. This loop brings you back within sight of the brick building. Return to the path in front of the structure, and follow it back toward the parking lot until you pass the marshy area and come to the hill. At the wooden post, go left 250 feet up the hill to the top, where you find a bench on your right with a great view of the marsh to your left.

Head downhill from here along the top of the small ridge, taking in great views of the marsh. The path follows a curve to the right along the edge of some oaks, and you come closest to the open water, though it is still a few hundred feet beyond the cattails. The last curve brings you around to the back of this ridge and the exit back to the trailhead and parking lot. Before you leave, check out the short mud trail right along the edge of the creek, left of the dock, which is popular for fishing and is a nice little foray into the cattails 100 feet from the parking lot. Also, on your way out of the park, you may see a trail into a small oak savanna restoration area on your left, just before you exit the park gate.

Nearby Activities

Cherokee Marsh North offers more hiking with a boardwalk and another view of the Yahara Watershed. Warner Park is at Sherman Avenue and WI 113 (Northport Drive), where you can catch a Madison Mallards baseball game during the summer. Check out their schedule online at **mallardsbaseball.com** or call 608-246-4277.

GPS COORDINATES AND DIRECTIONS
N43° 09' 11.99" W89° 23' 0.00"

Follow WI 113 (First Street) north from where it meets US 151 (East Washington Avenue). At the first traffic light, go right where it becomes East Johnson Street, but then follow the curve with Pennsylvania Avenue a block later. It becomes Packers Avenue 0.4 mile from there without leaving the main road, and finally it becomes Northport Road. Just be careful to follow the WI 113 signs. A total of 4 miles from US 151 at School Road, go right for three quarters of a mile. The park entrance is a small lot on your left. Pass through a gate here, set back 50 feet from the road, and continue down a gravel road 0.4 mile to the parking lot. The trailhead is to the left.

7 Edna Taylor Conservation Park

(WITH ALDO LEOPOLD NATURE CENTER AND WOODLAND PARK)

An observation platform at the water's edge—great for spying waterfowl

In Brief

The frogs take up the chorus and the birds have the melody at this symphonic wetland and forest nature preserve that abuts the Aldo Leopold Nature Center and Woodland Park, popular for school field trips and a goldmine for bird-watchers in the city.

Description

A glacial drumlin runs right down the middle of this park, and the trail rides its back. Edna Taylor was a teacher and dairy farmer who sold 37 of her 98 acres to Madison to help create this 56-acre conservation park. Sadly, she didn't live to see the completion of it.

The trail begins at the corner of the lot at a giant memorial stone dedicated to Edna Taylor. There are no facilities here except a trash can. The dirt and grass trail starts across prairie and savanna along the low ridge left by the last of the retreating glaciers. Grass will grow high on either side, and the path is flanked by marshland. This 1,000-foot length is unshaded. Cattails abound, and you can expect to see waterfowl (Canada geese and mallards are abundant), cranes, and herons. Flitting along the tops of the cattails are the usual redwing and tricolor blackbirds and the occasional kingbird (a blackbird whose breast and tip of the tail are white).

LENGTH & CONFIGURATION:
3.1-mile out-and-back with 3 loops
(plus 0.5-mile extra loop)

DIFFICULTY: Easy

SCENERY: Wetlands, oak forest,
savanna, ponds, interpretive trail

EXPOSURE: Half and half

TRAFFIC: Light to moderate

TRAIL SURFACE: Packed dirt, grass,
crushed stone, boardwalk

HIKING TIME: 1.5 hours

DRIVING DISTANCE: 1 mile from
the Beltline Highway (US 12/18) and
Monona Drive

ACCESS: 4 a.m.–1 hour after sunset

MAPS: USGS *Madison East;* artistic maps
on map boards near Aldo Leopold
Nature Center

WHEELCHAIR ACCESSIBILITY: Yes, in
most places. Wear gloves—there are a lot
of bird droppings in Aldo Leopold.

FACILITIES: Restrooms and water at
park office during business hours

CONTACT: **aldoleopoldnaturecenter.
org,** 608-221-0404; **cityofmadison.com/
parks**

COMMENTS: No dogs allowed. Report
park bird sightings at **ebird.org.** Find a
free kids trail guide PDF at the nature
center website. Kids should definitely
pick up the nature passport available at
the box at the turnaround outside the
nature center before starting. Hikers with
children may want to start their hikes
from the nature center.

At the other end of the pond, the brush closes in around the trail, with some oaks to your left. You might find raspberries here in July, but the park policy is no picking. Pass into the shade beyond this, where there's an enormous oak to your left. A patch of prairie to your right has a stunning array of wildflowers. The trail forks, and you need to go left; your return path brings you back here from the right. Pass into a very shaded oak forest with a crushed-rock path. Four hundred feet later, the trail opens up, and the sides slope into marshland. Cross a culvert here to find cottonwoods to the left and willows to the right. At the trail juncture, go left. This takes you beside a long pond on the right, with lily pads and blue-flag iris. The trail to the right exits the park in a residential neighborhood. Concrete blocks in the trail keep a low point from getting too muddy. Cattails stand on both sides. To your right, a big cottonwood stands right before the next pond. Now you have water on either side of you. Viewing platforms lean out into both ponds.

As the trail continues into smaller willows, pass under another oak. Then the trail opens to the sky as brush closes around you. The surface is packed dirt with roots and occasional rocks. You come out into a field as you exit Edna Taylor Park and enter Aldo Leopold Park through a line of evergreens. Signs make you aware of the change of parks.

Before you is a large pond with an island in the middle. Typically, you will find hordes of Canada geese here; if you come in spring, you'll see the tiny chicks. Geese can actually get aggressive, especially with young children who aren't much taller than the largest goose neck. The pond fills with tadpoles during this time, as well; not long after, the place comes alive with frog calls.

Edna Taylor Conservation Park
(with Aldo Leopold Nature Center and Woodland Park)

Canada Geese are common park visitors.

Use the wooden platforms along the edge of the pond to have closer looks at the water and to spot birds. Across the field, you can see the water towers of the Town of Monona inside Woodland Park. To continue on the trail, keep the pond to your left and follow the shoreline. You'll see the bridge to the island, and you might take a few moments to cross over and have a look around.

On the west side of the pond, trails go in many directions through the prairie and vary with park cutting. They provide access to plants in the middle of the fields and an educational trail that runs throughout Aldo Leopold Park. The trail leaves the water and passes along the park edge to the south. There are apartments beyond the line of mostly pine trees on your left.

The trail bends right near a stand of black walnut trees and passes along the prairie to a large mowed area with a picnic table and a wooden shed with a brick chimney to the left. Keep straight and come to a sign on the right welcoming you to Aldo Leopold Park. Here, there is a turnaround next to the nature center. A map box holds brochures and nature passports and includes information in Spanish. The nature center has restrooms, water, and park guides during business hours.

Continue along the left side of the road heading north past the turnaround and find another trailhead. Go left here as it cuts through the trees and brush, crosses the park entry road, and comes to a post marked WOODLAND TRAIL. Go left here through mowed grass on an unmarked path parallel to the road until you reach a map board that shows the layout of the Woodland Park trails. Go right, and the trail takes you into the woods and up the hill. You pass between the water towers and come to a trail juncture. Go left here on Morningside Trail. The trail loops out to Monona Drive, but rather than take the loop back, come around the bend and take a left down the Oak Savanna Trail. This will bring you around the edge of the park, reconnecting at the Woodland Trail, where you can see two American Indian mounds. Keep left and follow the short curve of the trail back around into the mowed area; follow that until it comes once again to the wooden post where you started. Retrace your steps across the road and back to the turn-around, where you rejoin the trail in Aldo Leopold Park.

From where you come back to the trail, go left and take the trail directly back to the pond. Go left and watch, as you walk along the pond, for a trail that cuts left across the prairie. Follow it to the park edge, where you pick up shade beneath the line of trees. Go right along the trail that curves back into the open in a small oak savanna, where you will find an informational sign regarding the savanna. Continue to the entrance of Edna Taylor Park, and go left, following your steps back through the ponds.

Beyond the ponds lies the trail to the left out of the park and the trail to the right from whence you came at the beginning of the hike. The next portion of the trail seems the most remote. Stay straight; don't duck back into the woods. Instead, follow another crushed-stone path with a long pond to your left. You have willows along this path and some cottonwoods to the right. Follow it 800 feet to the end of the pond, where there's a large culvert on the left. Just beyond that, the trail appears to end at a chain-link fence. From this gate, enter the back of the playground at Glendale Elementary School. Go right along the fence until the end of the mowed area, and the trail resumes going into thick woods on a packed-dirt trail.

The trail goes right at the next juncture before an enormous cottonwood. The left trail goes 0.3 mile up and over a hill but bypasses the upcoming boardwalk. It is also the end of an optional loop that would take you back through again what you are about to see.

Going right, you come to a narrow clearing on your left that runs to the top of the hill. Stay straight on the trail and come to a 250-foot boardwalk right through cattails as high as 6 to 8 feet above the boardwalk in some places. Open pond is about 20 feet off to your right. On the other side, the boardwalk extends onto dry land, ending at a packed-dirt trail full of rocks and roots. Oak trees tower over the low-lying underbrush.

The trail reaches another juncture as it comes into the open. Go right and follow the trail back to the original drumlin trail, where you go left back to the lot. If you go left here, you can take an additional 0.5 mile up and across a hill starting in oak savanna and then into thicker forest until it curves back down the hill and sends you back through the boardwalk section again.

Nearby Activities

The City of Monona has a public swimming pool at 1011 Nichols Road, no more than a 10-minute drive from here. Call 608-222-3098 for more information.

GPS COORDINATES AND DIRECTIONS
N43° 03' 6.45" W89° 19' 0.75"

From the Beltline Highway (US 12/18), go north on Monona Drive 0.6 mile and take a right on Femrite Drive. The parking lot for Edna Taylor is on the left 0.4 mile from Monona Drive. The trailhead is at the lot. (The entry to Aldo Leopold Nature Center is also on the left just 800 feet from Monona Drive.)

8 Elver Park

Children fish in the pond at the center of the park.

In Brief

Follow a prairie loop atop a hill overlooking Madison, and then explore the woods where an excellent disc-golf course is tucked among the trees.

Description

At 227 acres, this is the largest of Madison's community parks, and it seems there is always something going on here. Beginning from the first parking lot, look for the smaller pavilion closer to the park entrance. An asphalt path passes a playground and some tennis courts beyond the pavilion. Follow this as it leads you out toward the soccer field. At 0.15 mile, the asphalt curves toward the street and a crosswalk. Leave the path here and follow the edge of the cut grass as it curves behind the end of the soccer field and heads toward the bottom of the hill just 250 feet away. The trail becomes a wide mowed path and begins up the slope with trees and brush on either side until you reach the beginnings of prairie toward the top. It's 0.2 mile from the bottom to a trail juncture at the top. There are nice views of Madison behind you. Red-tailed hawks frequent this field, as do many songbirds. Going right will take you across the center of the prairie, but go straight. Three hundred feet later, on the left, is a spur trail out to the road and the local police station. Stay on the trail as it bends right, with brush gradually closing in around it. From the spur trail, it's

LENGTH & CONFIGURATION: 3.4-mile figure eight	**WHEELCHAIR ACCESSIBILITY:** Limited to a few paths around the open center of the park
DIFFICULTY: Easy to moderate	
SCENERY: Prairie, mixed forest, ponds, city skyline	**FACILITIES:** Restrooms, water, playground/splash park, shelter, picnic area
EXPOSURE: Half and half	**CONTACT:**
TRAFFIC: Light	**cityofmadison.com/parks/elver**
TRAIL SURFACE: Mowed grass, packed dirt, some asphalt	**COMMENTS:** Leashed dogs are allowed only below the sledding hill March 15–
HIKING TIME: 1.5 hours	November 15, but are not allowed on
DRIVING DISTANCE: 1.1 miles south of The Beltline Highway (US 12/14)	the trails. An outstanding disc-golf course offers an alternative trail starting from the
ACCESS: 4 a.m.–10 p.m. year-round	southeast corner of the ice-rink depression on the south side of the park. Little
MAPS: USGS *Middleton;* map board in ballpark parking lot	kids will enjoy Evler's splash park.

another 0.3 mile to the next juncture. Here a trail comes down the hill from your right. Continue straight and follow two fairways of the park's disc-golf course.

Another 0.2 mile brings you around a bend that slopes down a short distance and then rises up through some pines. A clearing runs from left to right, and you see a concrete pad (a golf "tee") to your left. Continue into the pines beyond the clearing and follow this trail, passing two trails that join at the same point on your right and finally arriving at a place where the wide path goes right and a narrow footpath plunges straight on into the forest. Take this and find a packed-dirt path that winds its way 0.3 mile down the hill, passing around a chain halfway down. If you are lucky, you may see an owl through here. (This is the most undeveloped segment of the park, and you can bypass it, if you prefer a groomed trail. Go right at the entry to the footpath and loop into the forest, and then follow the 17th-hole fairway to its end; then go left to head down the hill.)

From the bottom of the hill from either trail, go straight a bit farther until you come to the asphalt path and then follow that to the left. From the mapped trail, it is 0.2 mile to another juncture that goes right and crosses a bridge over the water to the ball diamonds. To your left is a nice bit of wetlands and a good place to find visiting birds during the migration periods. Go left along the asphalt path, which takes you to the north half of the park and will make a 1.6-mile loop through mixed forest back to the ballpark parking lot.

Into the woods 200 feet, the trail splits in two. These are one-way trails, coming and going, for skiers. For simplicity's sake, always take the left branch. Uphill 0.15 mile later, there is a spur footpath exiting the park to your left. Another 150 feet farther and around the bend, you come to another fork in the trail. Stay left and it's 0.25 mile to the next juncture, where you will find the parallel trail coming back to the right, plus two trails that lead directly right and would take you out toward the ballparks again. Just ahead is another fork;

Elver Park

ELVER PARK

Saalsaa Road
Hammersley Road
Jacobs Way
McKenna Boulevard
police department
To 18
Raymond Road
Gammon Lane
S. Gammon Road
To 12
Gammon Road
Mid Town Road
0.3 mile
0.2
0.1
0
0.3 kilometer
0.2
0.1
0
sports fields
High Point Road

stay left and hike 0.25 mile to the next multispoke juncture. Again, there's the parallel path behind you from the right, two paths that go slightly to the right ahead, and two more that go left. Take the trail to the left, which takes you on a 0.5-mile loop that will reconnect to the forward paths. Halfway up this loop is another meeting point of these parallel trails. Stay left once more. At the end of the 0.5-mile loop, go left and it's 0.2 mile more to exit the woods into the mowed area along the ballpark parking lot. You can follow the park road from here back to the other lot, or cross the lot and go to the corner of the nearest of the ball diamonds. From the beginning of the asphalt path, leave the asphalt and go on the grass trail toward the woods, passing the pond on your left and reaching another asphalt path. Follow this left back to the smaller pavilion and the parking lot.

This park is quite popular for its variety of activities. In the winter, there is ice skating as well as skiing, and the sledding hill is the best in town. Runners in training use that hill for an intense workout. This is also the site of the Fourth of July fireworks. Madison Metro bus routes 50 and 58 serve the park.

Nearby Activities

Vitense Golfland (608-271-1411, **vitense.com**), at 5501 West Beltline Highway at Whitney Way, can be reached by taking Schroeder Road heading east from Gammon Road (halfway back to the Beltline Highway from Elver Park). Here you'll find indoor/outdoor miniature golf, batting cages, a driving range, and a par 3 golf course.

GPS COORDINATES AND DIRECTIONS

N43° 02' 17.65" W89° 30' 10.15"

From The Beltline Highway (US 12/14), take the Gammon Road exit. Go left on Gammon Road/McKenna Boulevard 1.1 miles to the park entrance on the left. Park in the first lot on the left. The trailhead is at the southeastern corner of the lot near the smaller of two pavilions.

9 Lewis Nine Springs E-Way Trail

A view of wetlands from the end of the boardwalk

In Brief

Prairie and marsh along Spring Creek just south of Madison's Beltline Highway are home to wild turkeys, deer, and a variety of birds and wildflowers. Enter a world that seems much farther from the city than it is.

Description

The Lewis Nine Springs E-Way Trail is a 5.4-mile-long green corridor along the south side of Madison. The name honors Phil Lewis, a planner and professor at the University of Wisconsin who advocated strongly for the e-way. Laid out in 1970, it includes wetlands, farmland, and prairie and is an important part of the area's hopes for sustainable urban development and natural resource preservation. Part of the Capital City State Trail runs along its southern edge, and Lake Farm County Park and Capital Springs Centennial State Park and Recreation Area border it.

At the gravel parking lot, you'll find an accessible pit toilet, a self-pay tube, and a map board to the left of the trailhead. A larger kiosk is near the entrance to the parking lot

LENGTH & CONFIGURATION: 5.4 miles; a small loop within a large loop and a short out-and-back	**ACCESS:** 5 a.m.–10 p.m. year-round
	MAPS: USGS *Madison East;* at kiosk at trailhead
DIFFICULTY: Easy	
SCENERY: Prairie, wetlands, creek, some forest	**WHEELCHAIR ACCESSIBILITY:** Only the viewing platform and boardwalk
EXPOSURE: Mostly sun	**FACILITIES:** Accessible pit toilet, picnic tables
TRAFFIC: Light but moderate along the Capital City Trail segment	**CONTACT:** countyofdane.com/lwrd/parks/nine_springs.aspx
TRAIL SURFACE: Uneven cut grass, mowed paths, dirt, bridges, and boardwalk	**COMMENTS:** Hiking is not allowed when trails are maintained for skiing. Wild parsnip is common and shouldn't be touched (see Animal and Plant Hazards, page 12). There are daily fees for dogs and cross-country skiers, payable at the park.
HIKING TIME: 2–2.5 hours	
DRIVING DISTANCE: 1.1 miles from the Beltline Highway (US 12/18) and the South Towne Drive exit	

with more information about the greater park. A spur trail leads to a canoe launch on Lewis Nine Springs Creek.

Pass through a metal gate and come to a T intersection. Go left to explore the first loop, which amounts to a 0.6-mile hike through prairie to the highest point on the trail, where you have a modest view of the e-way and the surrounding city. In summer, you pass through rather tall grass, and the flowers throughout are impressive. Cross Spring Creek on a wooden bridge with railings (the canoe launch is to the left). Go left on the other side of the bridge, starting uphill through false sunflowers, yellow coneflowers, bergamot, and Queen Anne's lace. The trail follows the edge of a gentle hill. As it makes the curve, pass apple trees on the left and a short trail out to Lake Farm Road. You can cross over to the Lussier Family Heritage Center and Lake Farm County Park. The apple trees, of course, are beautiful in spring. Continue right and climb the hill on a moderate grade. At the top, you have a very nice view of the surrounding land all the way to the highway and of the marsh to the east. There are only a couple of trees near here; the rest is prairie laden with wildflowers.

Continue over the hump and find a bench and two wooden platforms, as well as a memorial plaque for Bud Morton, a champion for the e-way who called it Mother Nature's Bedroom. The trail that goes left from this clearing takes you 400 feet down to a dead end at the creek edge, or just before that you can take a 0.2-mile trail south to the paved Capital City State Trail. Explore if you wish; otherwise, go right from the bench and down the hill back to the bridge, and take the right branch from the trailhead.

The trail goes to the north edge of the e-way and heads west along the trees, which, later in the day, shade the trail. You have prairie to your left, but occasionally you pass in and out of clumps of trees and brush as you walk parallel to the creek. The trail is nicely cut

Lewis Nine Springs E-Way Trail

A fawn senses someone is watching from the park bench at the edge of a watering hole.

grass, unlike some of the field grass on the prairie loop, which is bristly and can be difficult to walk on, especially with sandals. After 0.5 mile, you come to a bridge over the creek.

Go right on the other side through high grass on a trail that goes straight along the creek. There is an abundance of birds here, from blackbirds to waterfowl. To the right beyond the marshy area, you can see a trailer court. At 0.4 mile, you reach a large bridge over the creek. If you continue straight, you enter an area with a brick building governed by Madison Metropolitan Sewerage District. The park has been trying to negotiate an easement for hikers to pass along the gravel road that connects this area to the Capital City State Trail at the intersection of Larsen Road and Clayton Road. If this happens, then you are looking at your return path for this hike. Some hikers pass through here anyway, but technically it is not allowed.

Cross the big bridge to your right and follow the path to the left into more prairie. Go under power lines as the trail puts prairie to your left and farmland to the right. From the bridge to the woods beyond the prairie is 0.4 mile, and you pass a line of box elders and a small clearing before the trees take over in earnest with shagbark hickory. The trail here is dirt, with twigs, sticks, roots, and mossy patches. Five hundred feet in, you find a bench on the right facing the trees. Another 500 feet brings you to another grassy trail out in the open, where you will find two ponds full of cattails. The trail goes around either side of the first one and then the second larger one as well, with a path that crosses between them. To the right of the second pond is a path out of the park to a residential neighborhood. Go to the end of these two ponds to behind the goal of a soccer field in Baxter Park.

Go left here as the trail slips back into the woods to the left of the soccer pitch and passes a lot of dead wood in a wet area before finding tall cottonwoods. The trail continues left into the woods, with houses along the perimeter to the right.

Now oaks enter the mix, smaller at first and then some larger ones. Much of the trail is cedar chip through here as it leads you into the area known as Indian Springs. Trails spur to the right out toward the neighborhood, and, 800 feet into the woods, there's a bench on the right at the head of one of these trails. Stay left and cross an 8-foot plank bridge over a ditch. Stay left once again as you pass a spur trail and come to a bench on the right overlooking a pond. This is a fine place to spy some local wildlife coming for a drink.

To your left, the trail goes around the pond, passing a clearing mowed to the creek's edge on your left. Come around the pond and arrive at a bridge to the left and a trail that leads straight out of the park to a turnaround at Anderberg Drive. That's a good place to park and then come right to this pond.

Cross the narrow railed bridge to the left and go left through the field along the creek to some trees where the trail heads right. Cross a field 400 feet and then go left (east). A spur trail at 500 feet doubles back and takes you along some birdhouses. Keep going straight 0.2 mile instead. You may find a trail that connects back to the trail you came in on, creating a lollipop; if so, you can follow this for your return trip. Otherwise, you can go right on a trail between two private agricultural fields along a row of tall trees. Follow it south 600 feet to the Capital City State Trail. This is asphalt, and you should go left here, following the multiuse trail 0.4 mile to the gravel road that goes left from the intersection of Larsen and Clayton Roads. Once the easement is granted, you can cross back to that bridge and go east back to the trailhead, retracing your steps. Until then, continue on this path 0.9 mile to the prairie trail on the left back into the e-way or 1.2 miles to Lake Farm Road to walk left 0.4 mile to the parking lot.

Be sure to check out the boardwalk into the marsh opposite the parking lot. A raised viewing platform 900 feet out gives nice views of waterfowl and eventually will be part of a more complete boardwalk trail.

Nearby Activities

Capital Springs State Recreation Park offers more trails through the marsh just across the street from the trailhead, as well as access to Lake Waubesa. The Capital City State Trail runs along the southern border of this trail and crosses the city to connect to other multiuse paths.

GPS COORDINATES AND DIRECTIONS

N43° 01' 51.44" W89° 20' 56.53"

Exit the Beltline Highway (US 12/18) at South Towne Drive and go south. This becomes Raywood Road. Go left 0.8 mile later on Moorland Road, continuing 0.3 mile to the trail parking lot on your right. The trailhead is at the southwest end of the lot.

10 Madison Capitol and Downtown

The view of the Capitol from State Street

In Brief

Stroll the eclectic downtown area, visit the majestic Capitol, climb Mansion Hill, and take in the lakeshores on both sides of the isthmus.

Description

Starting from the corner of Lake Street, begin up State Street toward the Capitol. Just about every style of ethnic food can be found in the next seven blocks (0.5 mile), from the classic Wisconsin State Street Brats to more exotic fare, such as Peruvian, Afghan, and Tibetan cuisines and Russian dumplings. Clothing, music, books, coffee shops, and an assortment of gift shops and boutiques make this a nice alternative to the usual mall-variety stores. Street musicians, university students, and a few panhandlers, unfortunately, are ubiquitous and add to the vibe that is quintessentially Madison.

You pass State Street Brats on your right halfway up the first block. Cross Gilman Street; in the next block to your left, across the street is Lisa Link Peace Park, where a historical marker remembers Madison's role in the antiwar movement in the 1960s and

LENGTH & CONFIGURATION: 3-mile loop	**ACCESS:** Year-round
DIFFICULTY: Easy	**MAPS:** USGS *Madison West*
SCENERY: Historical buildings, downtown shops, the Capitol, views of Lakes Mendota and Monona	**WHEELCHAIR ACCESSIBILITY:** Yes
	FACILITIES: In shops and restaurants along the route
EXPOSURE: Mostly sun	
TRAFFIC: Moderate to heavy	**CONTACT:** visitmadison.com
TRAIL SURFACE: Sidewalks	**COMMENTS:** This area is busiest on Saturday mornings, especially during Wisconsin Badger football games and the Farmers' Market.
HIKING TIME: 1 hour	
DRIVING DISTANCE: 0.5 mile from the Capitol Square	

1970s. Continue toward the Capitol and pass Sacred Feather, a fine hat store and one of the only freestanding houses along here. You'll cross the one-way, traffic-heavy Gorham Street and, another block later, Johnson Street heading the opposite direction. Henry Street crosses this intersection as well. Cross Johnson Street and then Henry Street to stay on State Street. At this corner, find the towering glass corner of the Madison Museum of Contemporary Art (closed Mondays; check **mmoca.org** or call 608-257-0158 for hours and exhibit information). There is a somewhat upscale rooftop terrace restaurant and bar. The view of State Street makes it worth a visit. The museum is part of the Overture Center for the Arts complex, which runs along the entire next block. Look for the old façades of two of the structures that once stood here—most notably the 1922 Capitol Theater; they were worked into the new building.

Across the street is the Orpheum Theatre, which brings in a mix of concert events throughout the year. In the last block of State Street before you reach the Capitol Square, find Ian's Pizza, a local favorite. At the top corner of State Street are two museums: The State Historical Museum and the Wisconsin Veterans Museum.

Cross the street to get to the Capitol at the corner of Mifflin and Carroll Streets. The Capitol is open to the public, free daily tours are available, and, from Memorial Day through October, you can climb to the observation deck for great views of the city in all directions. Hours are Monday–Friday 8 a.m.–6 p.m.; weekends and holidays 8 a.m.–4 p.m. Call 608-266-0382 for more information.

Go right along Carroll Street to Main Street, and head left. Halfway along the block is Martin Luther King (MLK) Jr. Boulevard. Go right here and follow it two blocks to get to the Monona Terrace. Based on a design by Frank Lloyd Wright, the convention center's rooftop terrace offers views of Lake Monona and occasional live music in the summer months.

Return along MLK Jr. Boulevard to the Capitol and continue around the square, going right on Main Street to Pinckney Street. Go left here and follow it to Mifflin Street. At this intersection, you will find the award-winning Madison Children's Museum

A corner market on State Street

(**madisonchildrensmuseum.org**). Cross Pinckney to the right and then Mifflin to the left, and take the angling Hamilton Street right and down the hill from the Capitol. You will walk three blocks (0.25 mile) to Gorham and cross to James Madison Park. This park along the shore of Lake Mendota offers canoe and sailboat rentals and is often alive with ultimate Frisbee, pickup basketball games, and sunbathers.

Go left and pass the 1863 Gates of Heaven synagogue, a sandstone and brick structure brought here from West Washington Avenue to be preserved. At Butler Street, go right one block and then left, climbing Gilman Street into what is known as the Mansion Hill District. Have a look at some fine houses from some of the wealthiest of the 19th-century Madisonians. After two blocks, go right on Wisconsin Avenue and come to the Edgewater Hotel, with its central terrace and bar overlooking Lake Mendota. Go left on Langdon Street and begin passing more rather large houses. Many of these are Greek fraternity or sorority houses. The Greek system began at the University of Wisconsin in 1857, and many of the chapter houses you see now were built in part as an answer to the housing problem before the advent of residence halls.

At the intersection of Carroll and Langdon Streets is a historical marker in honor of Frank Lloyd Wright and his relationship with the Madison area. You can follow Carroll Street to the lakeside, where steps lead you down for a view of the water. Continuing down Langdon Street, follow the street's bend to the right, and then continue two more blocks to Lake Street. Go right one short block to the end of the street, and follow the lakeside promenade to the left, which will take you to the University's Memorial Union Terrace. This is an excellent place to watch the sunset from the various tables and docks. Food and drink are available outdoors in season, and live musical acts are regularly scheduled on Thursday, Friday, and Saturday evenings. These events move indoors by late fall.

Heading away from the lakeside, cross through the parking lot with the Union to your right. On your left is an enormous redbrick building that looks more like a fortress. This is the 1893 Red Gym, which was once home to UW basketball and various other events.

Cross Langdon Street at the crosswalk in front of the Memorial Union, and take the angle walk through Library Mall that passes the central fountain. Just beyond that is a concrete speaker's pulpit. You can see the university's Chazen Museum of Art from here as well. Going left there will take you between the Memorial Library and University Bookstore and return you to your starting point at State and Lake Streets.

Nearby Activities

This is the heart of the Mad City, and activities are too numerous to list. The Dane County Farmers' Market on the Capitol Square on Saturday mornings from April through October is a Madison social event as much as a time to get local produce, cheese, meat, and baked goods. Another market is held off the square on Martin Luther King Jr. Boulevard on Wednesday mornings. Check out **visitmadison.com** for a calendar of other downtown events, such as Maxwell Street Days and Art Fair on the Square.

GPS COORDINATES AND DIRECTIONS
N43° 04' 29.11" W89° 23' 50.62"

From the Capitol Square, go northeast 0.2 mile (three blocks) on Wisconsin Avenue to Gorham Street. Go left and follow Gorham 0.4 mile as it crosses State Street and bends right, becoming University Avenue. Two blocks later, turn right on Lake Street and park in the parking ramp half a block down on the right. The hike begins another half block beyond at the corner of Lake and State Streets.

11 Olin Park and Turville Point Conservation Park

The view from Olin Park across Lake Monona toward the Capitol

In Brief

Venture out to Turville Point jutting into Lake Monona, take a tour through the woods and a bit of prairie, and have a picnic with a view of the Capitol.

Description

From the trailhead, start straight for the woods to a grassy trail into oak savanna. Through the trees to the left is Lake Monona. Pick up a packed-dirt trail and come to a sign that reads CONSERVATION PARK-TURVILLE POINT. Pass through a gate and, at the first trail juncture, go left on a dirt footpath. Brush thickens into the savanna as you go. Just 200 feet along the trail, a spur trail breaks left from the main trail. Take it to the water's edge where basswoods dangle their leaves into the lake. The trail is uneven here, with tree roots and strewn branches and twigs. This spur lasts only 0.1 mile before curving to the right and rejoining the main path again. There isn't much difference in length, but being closer to the lake is nicer.

Go left at the connection; the trail curves gently toward the lake again as it heads downhill. The trail is roughly maintained; a mower puts a wide cut through the brush on either side of the path, and it is not grassy. Pass a narrow footpath spur trail to the right at

LENGTH & CONFIGURATION: 2-mile loop within a loop	**ACCESS:** 4 a.m.–1 hour after sunset
DIFFICULTY: Easy	**MAPS:** USGS *Madison East*
SCENERY: Mixed forest, Lake Monona, the Capitol, a small prairie	**WHEELCHAIR ACCESSIBILITY:** None
EXPOSURE: Mostly shaded	**FACILITIES:** Restrooms, water, shelter, picnic area
TRAFFIC: Light	**CONTACT:** www.cityofmadison.com/parks/parks/park.cfm?id=1361
TRAIL SURFACE: Packed dirt, stones, and tree roots; some mowed paths	
HIKING TIME: 45 minutes–1 hour	**COMMENTS:** No dogs allowed. This trail is good for runners who like a little challenge. The loops through the oak savanna and prairie are best; some may not prefer the occasional roots along the other trails.
DRIVING DISTANCE: 1.2 miles from John Nolen Drive and the Beltline Highway (US 12/18)	

200 feet. Then the trail bends to the right into a hollow. Heading slightly uphill, the path breaks from the lake on crushed rock and then descends again. You can see water through the trees both on the left and right as you head out onto Turville Point. The trail breaks left at a right angle and heads straight toward water, where it curls around the edge of the point. There have been reports of osprey and bald eagles out here, and you get a view of sky as you round the point. Cattails grow along the lake edge, and a short spur trail goes out onto the rocks at the very tip of the point.

From the rocks to the next spur trail is 0.25 mile. The trail heads south along the point with the lake on the left. The earth is typically damp as it runs close to the waterline and even below it at times. You can hear the Beltline Highway (US 12/18) from here. The path bends right and heads easily uphill and away from water. As you climb, the land slopes to the left. The tree coverage is primarily black walnut. Crest the hill at the cutoff path that bears right. Stay left through a small dip in the trail and up another slope.

Where the trail levels off, you find views out over the lake in spring and fall. Descend on the other side on a crushed-rock surface with occasional wood beams to prevent erosion. The path skirts the lakeshore one more time. During the hot summers, the lake can get quite green, and the smell might deter some from the area.

The trail passes along the water's edge again after 0.15 mile and then heads to the right away from water. Pass a spur trail to the left out to a commercial zone outside the park. The trail continues gently uphill for 0.2 mile through a scattering of acorns, walnuts, and hickory nuts. You can expect a nice selection of woodland wildflowers along here. The trail forks at 0.2 mile, the left trail continuing on the outer loop. Go right here and cross a woodland trail coming from your right (that previous connector path from the lakeside), and then step into a large clearing in the middle of the conservation park. This is a prairie restoration area. Go left and follow the 0.4-mile looping trail through native grasses and wildflowers around the clearing back to this point again. If you want to shorten this hike, continue out the other side of the prairie and take a trail past a chain, and then cross straight through the oak

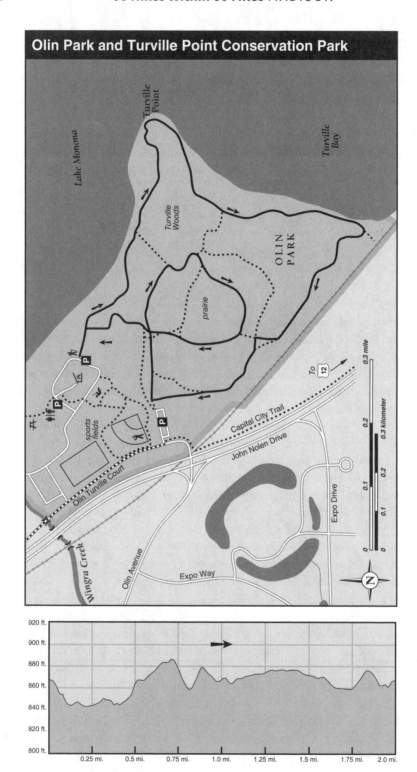

savanna to the parking area. Otherwise, when you finish the prairie loop and come back to the trail juncture where you entered it, go right as you head back into the woods. The trail will follow along the top of a ridge that drops about 20 feet down on your left and looks out over the railroad tracks and John Nolen Drive beyond that.

At 0.1 mile from the juncture, the trail turns to the right away from the edge and starts to head downhill as it bends around the hill that the prairie is resting on. An alternative trail heads to the right up along the edge of the prairie. Stay left and pass a trail exit to a different parking lot to the left, just before you arrive at a T at a concrete access road. Go uphill to the right with oak savanna to the left.

At 0.1 mile, many trails intersect. Just to your left is that chain, beyond which is the oak savanna between you and the parking lot. This is an option, with trails going along the perimeter in either direction or at an angle right over the gentle hill. A trail to the right takes you out into the prairie loop, and another trail goes straight through the woods parallel to the prairie trail. Look for a trail on your left that passes between the two wooden posts of a gate in the conservation park fence. The narrow footpath skirts to the right of the oak savanna and passes 0.1 mile through the woods back to the first trail juncture on this hike. The path to the left takes you back out of the park and across the lawn to the parking lot.

Nearby Activities

The Capital City Trail follows an asphalt path from the north end of the park 1.1 miles across Monona Bay and along the lakeshore. This takes you to the Monona Terrace Community and Convention Center (**mononaterrace.com**), which is based on a design by Frank Lloyd Wright.

GPS COORDINATES AND DIRECTIONS
N43° 03' 13.17" W89° 22' 29.73"

From the Beltline Highway (US 12/18), go north on John Nolen Drive 0.7 mile to the Olin Avenue intersection. Go right on Olin Turville Court as it runs parallel to John Nolen Drive. Follow this 0.25 mile to the park entrance and go right. Follow the park road 0.25 mile and stay right as it takes a turn around the pavilion at the top of the hill. To the southeast of the pavilion along the road is a small perpendicular parking area. The trail is at the lakeside corner of the lot.

12 Owen Conservation Park

Professor Owen's former retreat is now a conservancy with a view.

In Brief

One of Madison's best-kept secrets, the prairie here offers an overlook to the city that shows only a fraction of the buildings and gives the illusion that there is nothing around you but forest.

Description

Just the fact that this used to be a farm should give you an idea of how much Madison has grown over the years. On a hilltop overlooking Madison's west side, this 93-acre park was once the summer retreat of former university professor Edward T. Owen. He called it Torwald. A professor of French, Owen feared that reckless urban development would spoil the natural beauty of Madison. With colleagues John Olin and Edward Hammersley, he donated land for a 12-mile pleasure drive on the west side. Today, prairie and oak savanna have reclaimed the park. Coneflower, goldenrod, bluestem, and many other prairie flowers and grasses create a sea of waving colors in the growing season. Various entry paths from all sides give the place a neighborhood-park accessibility, but the tall trees around its perimeter give the illusion that much of the surrounding world is undeveloped.

The loop around the central prairie is a common evening promenade for locals, but this hike includes a segment through the surrounding woods on a narrow footpath as

LENGTH & CONFIGURATION: 1.5-mile loop	**ACCESS:** 4 a.m.–1 hour after sunset
DIFFICULTY: Easy, with some moderate	**MAPS:** USGS *Madison West;* on map board
SCENERY: Mixed woods, prairie, city skyline overlook	**WHEELCHAIR ACCESSIBILITY:** None
EXPOSURE: Shaded and sun	**FACILITIES:** Restrooms, drinking fountain
TRAFFIC: Light	**CONTACT:** www.cityofmadison.com/ parks/parks/park.cfm?id=1305
TRAIL SURFACE: Packed dirt, grass, wood chip	**COMMENTS:** No dogs or bikes allowed. Trails are groomed for skiing in winter. Listed at **ebird.org** as a birding hot spot. Madison Metro bus routes 8 and 15 serve the park.
HIKING TIME: 1 hour	
DRIVING DISTANCE: 1.1 miles west of University Avenue and Whitney Way	

well. The forest features an assortment of wildflowers more suited to shade and a varying topography that recalls what the west side must have looked like before development.

There is a map board in the parking lot with an aerial-view photograph of the park with the trails highlighted. Look for the trailhead in the northwest corner of the parking lot to the left of the restrooms.

A grassy trail heads uphill and immediately hits a juncture. Go right and pass a padlocked wooden door into a stone wall that resembles a cellar. The path is narrow, just wide enough for one's feet. Expect a lot of tree roots as this 0.2-mile loop rounds the hill in this corner of the park. To the right, the land slopes down. It rises above you to the left and is shaded by maples. Pass along a stone wall on your left midway around the hill. Throughout this section, watch for Virginia broadleaf and columbine.

The trail splits, but the two paths—the low road and the high road, you might say—run parallel a short distance, passing another stone wall and a trailside bench and coming back together soon after. At the next fork in the trail, go right. There are more wood beams laid here in the trail, so watch for them because grasses start to lean over the already narrow trail, sometimes preventing you from seeing where you are stepping.

At the next juncture, stay left. Right takes you out of the park. You come to another park bench where the trail begins to rise a bit and wildflowers are prominent. The trail curves left, but head right at the next trail. The left trail returns in the direction you came from.

Pass through an area thick with wildflowers and reach a four-way trail juncture. Left takes you to the parking lot, and right leads you out of the park. Go straight and enter the prairie. Once you're there, wood chips cover the trail to the right, which eventually gives way to mowed grass. Trails crisscross the open prairie to the left. The view here is amazing, with only the tallest landmarks puncturing the green of Madison.

Pass a trail on your left, continuing on an easy grade to the bottom of the hill with the trees to your right. As you come to oak savanna, the trail bends left to cross the southern end of the park.

Owen Conservation Park

The forest on your right draws back about 100 feet. As you cross the field, you come into the shade again of an oak tree. A trail goes right, where you can find some small loops through the trees and three exit trails to the surrounding residential areas. A couple of ponds back here may offer some waterfowl viewing from time to time.

Brush thickens on the left, blocking the field to the north from view in green seasons. The canopy over the trail opens to the sky, just as the trail starts its turn north up the opposite side of the center of the prairie/savanna. The trail takes you through open and shaded patches. There is a bench at the trail that cuts back across the savanna, and another trail goes right into the trees and out to residences. You'll find a similar trail juncture 300 feet from here and another 300 feet beyond that, which would take you left to the parking lot.

Keep going straight and uphill. Grasses can grow taller than 6 feet here. The trail makes an easy 0.3-mile semicircle along the edge of the forest, taking you across the northern portion of the prairie. There is a lot of intervening brush to your left. As the trail heads west and starts to bend south for the return, you see that where you are walking is lower than the hump of the central prairie. The land slopes down to the right into the forest. You reach the edge of the park road, where a gate offers an entry point to the trail that is before the parking lot, which is nice if you enter the park on foot.

At the next trail juncture, a branch goes to the parking lot to the right. You can observe a row of trees to your left that goes directly across the prairie, dividing it with another alternative trail.

Trilliums and wild geraniums are abundant in the spring. Be aware that the park often administers springtime burns as part of the efforts to restore the prairie by eliminating invasive plants. You can call the Madison Parks Division at 608-266-4711 to find out if there was a burn.

Nearby Activities

In 1890, two of Owen's children died during a diphtheria epidemic. Two boulders on Regent Street, just west of the Speedway Road and Highland Avenue intersection, commemorate them and mark Owen Drive, a pleasure drive Professor Owen donated to the city in their names. Take a bit of the pleasure drive by following Regent Street west from here, where it becomes Owen Drive as it passes through Hoyt Park to connect with Mineral Point Road.

GPS COORDINATES AND DIRECTIONS
N43° 04' 22.42" W89° 29' 15.36"

From its intersection with University Avenue on the west side, follow Whitney Way south 0.2 mile to Old Middleton Road. Go right (west) 0.6 mile to Old Sauk Road. Turn left; at 0.4 mile, the park entrance is on your left. Follow the park road to the parking lot. The trailhead is to the right of the lot entry in the northwest corner of the lot.

13 Pheasant Branch Conservancy

(WITH PHEASANT BRANCH CREEK TRAIL)

The view from Frederick's Hill

In Brief

An outstanding conservancy project that features a little bit of everything: a stunning view of Madison and the Capitol, restored prairie and wetlands, a big spring, and a mixed-forest hike along a creek that crosses back and forth over the trail in six places.

Description

The village of Pheasant Branch was a stagecoach stop back in 1847, near what is now Century Avenue. The Stamm House, where travelers might spend the night or get a bite to eat, is still there and serving. Much of what is here today, preserved in the conservancy, was once converted to farmland. As Middleton grew and developed land, the runoff water also increased. The little Pheasant Branch Creek became overwhelmed and started putting too much sediment into Lake Mendota. The municipality rerouted the creek a bit

LENGTH & CONFIGURATION: Up to 7.6 miles; loop and out-and-back	**ACCESS:** 7 a.m.–10 p.m.
DIFFICULTY: Easy, with one moderate climb	**MAPS:** USGS *Middleton* and *Madison West;* posted map boards
SCENERY: Prairie, oak savanna, wetlands, mixed forest, running water, springs	**WHEELCHAIR ACCESSIBILITY:** Yes
	FACILITIES: Restrooms, water, vending machine
EXPOSURE: Shade and sun	**CONTACT: pheasantbranch.org/direc-tions.html**
TRAFFIC: Moderate	
TRAIL SURFACE: Crushed rock, boardwalk, packed dirt, stepping-stones	**COMMENTS:** Leashed dogs allowed. The Pheasant Branch Trail portion requires you to use stepping-stones to cross five concrete "bridges" submerged in the ankle-deep creek. There are numerous optional entry points to the trail system; see parking lots on the map.
HIKING TIME: 3 hours	
DRIVING DISTANCE: 1 mile from the intersection of County Roads M and Q in Middleton	

in 1970, through the marshes you see today, so that much of that sediment and the pollutants in the runoff can be filtered before the creek empties into the lake.

From the Orchid Heights Park trailhead, start south on asphalt through a pleasant recreational park. To your right, you can see ponds and marshland popular for migrating birds in the spring and fall. The path is shared with bicyclists, and there is no shade through here. At 500 feet, pass a transformer station. Beyond this, the field is not mowed. You see oaks to the left and prairie to the right. Watch for hawks and field birds.

Stay on the trail to the right at the first intersection and find a crushed-rock trail. You reach a line of trees and another trail juncture. A trail goes straight, up a hill toward a water tower, and out of the park 0.3 mile to the south on Highland Way. Go right, with trees to your right and prairie to your left, and follow the edge of the field as it bends south and enters mixed woods at 500 feet.

The path is shaded and the understory is waist-high, allowing you to see deep into the woods to the left. Pass a bench on your left, and, 0.3 mile from where you entered the shade, come out again, with houses up on the ridge to the left. Shade is limited to a few box elders and cottonwoods along the path. You reach a bridge over Pheasant Branch Creek at another 0.3 mile. From here it breaks from the residential zone and, 200 feet later, joins a boardwalk wide enough for bikes, pedestrians, and two-way traffic. A spur trail cuts right through a wooden fence 500 feet farther along and leads to a platform overlooking the marsh, where you may see wood ducks, mallards, herons, and sandhill cranes.

The boardwalk ends just 300 feet from this spur trail, and another trail 200 feet after that bears left out to Century Avenue. Neither spur trail allows bikes or dogs. You come to a trail intersection with a bench to your right. Now you have a choice. The trail straight across the bridge before you and the one to the left are essentially the same and connect on the other side of the creek. (The one to the right allows bikes.) Choose these to skip

Pheasant Branch Conservancy (with Pheasant Branch Creek Trail)

the creek trail. The trail to the left leads out to Century Avenue, where there is a trail kiosk with history and other information, a couple of restaurants, and a gas station for refreshments and restrooms. This is also the connection to the Pheasant Branch Creek Trail, which makes a 3-mile out-and-back segment of this 7.6-mile hike. Skip ahead if you are skipping the creek trail.

Pheasant Branch Creek Trail Go left 0.3 mile to the park entrance on Century Avenue. Cross at the traffic lights at Branch Street and Century Avenue to your left. Go right (west), cross the bridge over the creek, and enter Pheasant Branch Nature Preserve. Bikes and dogs are permitted here as well. There's a map board on the right and water on the left. Cross the creek five times on concrete stepping-stones. Bicycles ride through several inches of water that flow over each concrete "bridge."

The trail is partly shaded by black walnuts and oaks, and you can see the creek flowing toward you, tumbling over rocks. The trail curves right and opens up in a hollow with houses tucked back in woods on either side. The trail comes to a dip and your first crossing at 0.2 mile with a dozen steps across a 20-foot concrete creek bed. Five hundred feet later, the trail crosses the creek again. On the other side of the creek, a small meadow opens under the trees. The trail bends gently to the right, and 0.2 mile from this crossing is the next. The trail climbs the last 100 feet to street level. A sign marks the entrance near a service gate, and there's a map of the trail. Cross Park Street; the trail continues on the other side, where you'll see two giant storm sewers to the right. Left is a marshy area, and a bench is to your right.

Just 0.4 mile from Park Street is the next creek crossing, and the final crossing is another 500 feet after that.

Just on the other side of the creek, wood-beam-and-dirt steps lead up to the back of Middleton Alternative High School. Continuing past the steps, the path becomes asphalt and takes you either left up to Parmenter Street or straight under the overpass of the Old Beltline Highway to more groomed trails at Confluence Pond, Deming Way, Northern Fork Trail, and even out past Middleton Airport. This is the turnaround for this hike, and you must retrace your steps back across Century Avenue, into the conservancy once again, to the trail intersection with the bridge over the creek.

Conservancy Trail Back at that juncture with the creek trail, the bridge to your left (west) is foot traffic only and follows a narrow boardwalk; bikes follow the trail north along the creek and cross a bigger bridge before rejoining the other trail. Cross the bridge and follow the boardwalk as it takes a right-angle right turn and then meets the main trail again. Go left here and see condos up the slope before you. The crushed-stone path is wider and exposed. At the next T-intersection, go right. The trail left leads out of the park to the condos.

From here the path runs straight, and at 0.2 mile there is a trail left and up the hill to the parking lot, where there is a nice overlook of the park and a bench to enjoy it from. Go straight if you don't want to take the hill.

From the parking lot, a paved bike trail follows the road north, but go right on the footpath through savanna. The trail descends sharply and connects again to the main trail. Go left to find the end of the asphalt trail from the lot and a gate in front of you. Go right along Pheasant Branch Road for 0.3 mile, passing more parking and crossing a small footbridge over a swampy area at 500 feet.

Then the trail cuts right at 90 degrees from the road, and it continues through prairie, crossing a bridge and taking you 0.2 mile to a trail juncture. To the right is an informational kiosk, and to the left is another parking area/trailhead along Pheasant Branch Road. Straight ahead takes you 0.6 mile back to the parking lot, and a soft right leads down a short slope to a lower level of prairie and marsh.

Go left up the moderately steep mowed-grass path that takes you 1 mile on a path that goes up along the slope of Frederick's Hill around the back to the top. From that point, the trail does a loop through oak trees around the crown of the hill. Starting left on the loop, come to a wonderful scenic overlook and a bench. From here you can see all the way to the Capitol in downtown Madison. Backtrack to where you left the main trail, and notice there is a small network of trails around the hill area. When you return to the kiosk area, look for that sloping trail down to another level. Take that path, rather than the main trail, 800 feet to an observation platform, where you can see spring water bubbling up through the sandy soil in a small pool.

From the platform, go right up the hill to rejoin the main trail. Pass another information kiosk immediately on your right, and it's just another 0.4 mile along the crushed-rock path back to the parking lot.

Nearby Activities

Capital Brewery in Middleton offers tours and hosts a beer garden on summer evenings. Check them out at **capital-brewery.com** or call 608-836-7100.

GPS COORDINATES AND DIRECTIONS
N43° 07' 7.37" W89° 28' 38.42"

From the intersection of CR M and CR Q in Middleton, go north 0.4 mile on CR Q to Rolling Hill Drive and turn left. Take the first right 300 feet later on Larkspur Road. Follow this to its end, less than 0.2 mile, and turn right on Valley Ridge Road. Go 500 feet and take the first left on Sedge Meadow Road. Cross two speed bumps and take the first left, which is the entrance to the parking lot at Orchid Heights Park. The trailhead is at the map board near the restrooms.

14 Picnic Point

A view of the Capitol from University Bay

In Brief

Stroll along the shores of Lake Mendota, see the university, and find the best view of the Capitol from across the water.

Description

There is perhaps no more famous strolling destination in Madison than Picnic Point. This narrow peninsula into Lake Mendota is a magnet for nature lovers, joggers, and the hopelessly romantic. The trail runs the length of the University of Wisconsin–Madison's Lakeshore Nature Preserve, which protects this beautiful portion of Lake Mendota from development, preserving it for ecological and environmental study, as well as pure aesthetics.

Also referred to as the Lakeshore Path, it has two parts: the more popular eastern portion, the Howard Temin Lakeshore Path, which runs from the university to Picnic Point, and the Lake Mendota Lakeshore Path, which starts at Picnic Point and heads west. The latter is open only to foot traffic, while the former is shared with bicyclists in many places. Altogether, it makes the most beloved walk in the city, enjoyed by residents, students, and visitors alike.

The trailhead is located just past the docks at the terrace behind the Memorial Union at the University of Wisconsin. Look for a gravel path right behind the Arthur D. Hasler Lab of Limnology. The trail shows high traffic, as many students, joggers, and bicyclists pass through here.

LENGTH & CONFIGURATION: 8-mile two-way out-and-back	**ACCESS:** The preserve opens at sunrise and closes at 10 p.m.
DIFFICULTY: Easy, but moderate west of Picnic Point	**MAPS:** USGS *Madison West;* interactive and printable maps online
SCENERY: Lake Mendota, mixed forest, and views of the Capitol and the university	**WHEELCHAIR ACCESSIBILITY:** From the trailhead to Picnic Point but not the trail segment beyond
EXPOSURE: Mostly shaded, with some open stretches	**FACILITIES:** Restrooms on the trail and back at the Memorial Union
TRAFFIC: Heavy along campus, moderate toward the point, light beyond the point	**CONTACT:** lakeshorepreserve.wisc.edu
TRAIL SURFACE: Crushed rock, packed dirt, some asphalt	**COMMENTS:** Leashed dogs allowed; bicycles limited to designated areas. If you are only seeking Picnic Point, park nearby along University Bay Drive at parking lots 129 or 130; it is 0.9 mile to the point itself.
HIKING TIME: 2.5–3 hours	
DRIVING DISTANCE: From University Avenue and Park Street, go north 2 blocks to reach the trailhead.	

Just over 100 feet in on your right is a park bench and a good lookout point out over the water to your halfway point and the trail's namesake, as well as a staircase down from campus to your left. The trail skirts the lake's edge 5–15 feet above the water level throughout this section, offering plenty of shade and views out onto the water.

In another 500 feet, pass another trail coming down from the left via Muir Woods. Just past this is an emergency phone and an access road coming down the hill also on your left. On your right side is a viewing platform under a weeping willow; trail users sometimes lock their bikes here. Beyond here, 900 feet on the left and up a few stairs, is one of the university permit-only parking lots.

Once you pass this, the trail opens up to the lawn behind some dormitories. Students lounge here studying, sunbathing in between trees, or simply escaping for a moment.

The building coming up on your left is Porter Boathouse, where the UW crew teams keep their boats. When they are moving shells in and out of the boathouse, gates close on the path and all trail traffic is diverted around the back of the building for that short stretch.

An asphalt bike path joins the trail and the hiking trail runs alongside it until Lot 126 on your right, about 1,300 feet past the boathouse. This lot requires a permit Monday–Friday from 7 a.m. to 4:30 p.m. Cross the entrance to the lot and look for the hiking trail as it descends to the right and becomes a narrow path of packed dirt running at a level 5 feet lower than the bike trail. This is Willow Creek Woods, and the trail runs 500 feet through it before rising up to join the bike path again and cross the bridge over the creek itself. After this, foot traffic stays right, and the bikes have their own separate strip of asphalt. Exposure from here is partly shaded, because the trail passes beneath one willow

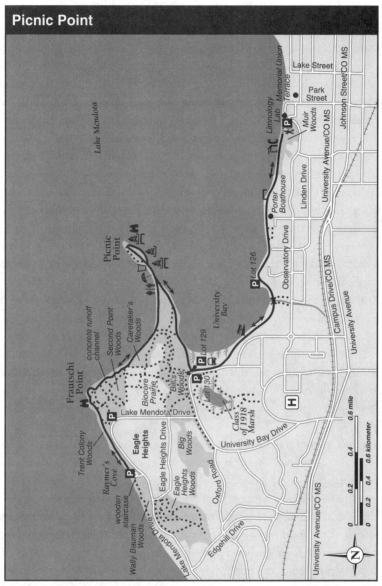

Picnic Point

Lake Street

Park Street

Johnson Street/CO MS

Lake Memorial Union

Terrace

Limnology Lab

Muir Woods

P

Lake Mendota

Porter Boathouse

Linden Drive

Observatory Drive

University Avenue/CO MS

Campus Drive/CO MS

Lot 126

P

Picnic Point

University Bay

Second Point Woods

Caretaker's Woods

concrete runoff channel

Lot 129

P P

University Avenue

Frauschi Point

M

Biocore Prairie

Bill's Woods

Lot 130

P

Class of 1918 Marsh

H

P

Lake Mendota Drive

Trent Colony Woods

Eagle Heights

Eagle Heights Drive

Big Woods

University Bay Drive

Raymer's Cove

P

Eagle Heights Woods

Oxford Road

0.6 mile

wooden staircase

Wally Bauman Woods

Lake Mendota Drive

Edgehill Drive

0.6 kilometer

0   0.2   0.4

0   0.2   0.4   0.6

University Avenue/CO MS

N

920 ft.
900 ft.
880 ft.
860 ft.
840 ft.
820 ft.
800 ft.

0.5 mi.   1.0 mi.   1.5 mi.   2.0 mi.   2.5 mi.   3.0 mi.   3.5 mi.   4.0 mi.

or basswood tree after another until you reach a boat landing 0.25 mile away. Beyond this, there is no shade until you enter the gates of Picnic Point another 0.4 mile beyond that.

Throughout this stretch, University Bay is on your right. Redwing blackbirds bob atop cattails, over which is a view of the Capitol. Painted turtles cross from here to Class of 1918 Marsh inland to your left. This segment from the bridge to the stone gate is a good place to see migratory birds in season. In fact, the marsh across the street has its own little loop trail popular with birders. Beyond all this, to your left, is the sprawling University Hospital.

Lot 129, just outside the entrance to the point, has a three-hour limit. From 7 a.m. to 4:30 p.m. you must pay at the parking terminal. Lot 130 is across the street near the marsh trail. These parking lots are good starting points for anyone looking to cut out the busiest portion of the trail close to the university or simply take the short walk out to Picnic Point directly (1.8 miles round-trip). The bus stop here is served by the free route 80 bus, which runs from Eagle Heights to the Memorial Union.

The entrance to the Picnic Point section of the preserve is through a gate in a stone wall next to the parking lot, where there is also a map of the entire park. Just inside the gate, a trail cuts left to Eagle Heights, but follow the trail to the right along the eastern shore of the point. Short paths through the trees and underbrush on your right grant clear views across the lake.

The clearing shows mowed lawn to the left, a nice spot for picnics or taking a break in the sun. This lawn tapers and ends where the trail again enters the trees about 800 feet from the park entrance. Just past this is a cutoff trail to the left, which leads directly to the next segment of the trail and bypasses the point itself.

Continuing on, an area under the trees opens up to accommodate two fire pits to your right.

Look for stacks of free firewood along the path. It is provided to help protect the park from the emerald ash borer, an invasive insect species that travels with firewood from outside a region.

A small beach 0.2 mile later on your left is The Narrows, the thinnest point on the peninsula. Just past here, the trail splits from the main. Follow along to the right on a packed-dirt path for another 0.2 mile until you reach Picnic Point. There are three more fire pits along this stretch and a water pump on your left just 200 feet past the beach. The fountain portion of this water pump (known as a "bubbler" as drinking fountains are often called in Wisconsin) is specially designed with a reservoir so that you don't have to keep pumping to take a sip.

The point is another small clearing, and there are side paths down to the water's edge that will give you better views of the city after the leaves have come in during spring. The point also has a fire pit and a bench with a view; however, in summer the view is mostly obscured by foliage.

As you return, look for the narrow trail to the right, which follows the western side of the peninsula and looks down over the slope to the water a bit before rejoining the main trail again at The Narrows and the beach. Stay right, and again veer west down another narrow path. Restrooms with pit toilets are 200 feet down on your left. Just beyond this, look for the two largest trees, a pair of basswoods out on the point.

This segment is really quite different from the rest of the trail, and many visitors to the point have never even explored it. The trail becomes a mix of packed dirt and sand, and the city seems very far away. You enter a marshy area where the noise of the frogs overpowers the volume of the birds. Six hundred feet beyond this is an abandoned shelter house and the other end of the cutoff trail you passed heading out to the point. Stay right here.

The trail becomes more challenging past this point, rising and falling and given over to exposed roots and rocks. It breaks from the shore and heads inland to Biocore Prairie, the result of a restoration project in 1997. The trail skirts along the corner before ducking back into the woods.

About 200 feet in, cross an old concrete water channel with a gate. Just beyond this is the entrance to Second Point Trail. Stay right along the shoreline. Another trail branching off to the left 400 feet beyond this would take you to the parking lot or deeper into North Shore Woods.

Coming up on your right is a scenic viewpoint to the lake at Frautschi Point. From here pass through Tent Colony Woods, where, from 1912 to 1962, as many as 300 graduate students would set up wall tents and live with their families for the summer. When you reach the parking lot 0.5 mile past the point, look for a wooden staircase down to the right to Raymer's Cove. Go here to get down to the water's edge and see the sandstone cliffs. This is particularly nice at sunset.

If you are too tired to do the return trip, the free route 80 bus stops at Eagle Heights across Lake Mendota Drive from the parking lot. It will take you all the way back to the Memorial Union. This lot is also a nice starting point for an out-and-back hike, or you can arrive here by bus and take the trail one-way to downtown.

Nearby Activities

The Memorial Union attracts not just students but Madisonians of all ages to take in the views, enjoy a drink or burger on the lovely lakeside terrace, and listen to live music on weekends in seasonable weather. Try some of the University of Wisconsin's own ice cream inside. The Capitol is a 10-minute walk from here up State Street, the city's liveliest strip of shops, coffee shops, and restaurants.

GPS COORDINATES AND DIRECTIONS

N43° 04' 38.02" W89° 24' 11.37"

From University Avenue downtown, turn right onto Lake Street and park in the ramp on your right. Walk to the end of Lake Street and follow it left past the Memorial Union Terrace to reach the trailhead.

15 Pope Farm Park

A stone wall alongside the trail

In Brief

Learn about the glaciers as well, as American Indian and pioneer agriculture, as you climb a couple of recessional moraines of prairie and farmland offering views all the way to Madison's Capitol dome.

Description

With urban development seemingly racing west from Madison, how fortunate it is that the Pope family of the town of Middleton has set aside this 105-acre park that is partly a working farm. The view of the Madison Capitol in the distance alone makes this park worth a visit, but as you walk the top of two moraines, you take in prairie and farmland with some great educational signage along the way. Rhyolite present in the stone fence that climbs the hill is evidence of the tremendous earth-moving of the glaciers of the Ice Age. The closest regional deposit of this stone is in the Lake Superior basin.

The trail system includes color-coded paths of varying lengths (0.45–1.9 miles) and varied terrain, but the route outlined here combines them to give you a nice overview of the park. The trail starts up the hill along the edge of a stone fence on your left. You pass prairie restoration on your way up. At 750 feet, you reach parking for the scenic overlook, where there are a couple of portable toilets. Just past this are two simple amphitheaters to the right, fashioned with sitting stones and several educational signs. The view east is all the way to the dome just over 9 miles away.

LENGTH & CONFIGURATION: 2.5-mile loop	**ACCESS:** Sunrise to sunset
DIFFICULTY: Easy, some moderate	**MAPS:** USGS *Middleton;* on signs at trailheads and several trail junctures
SCENERY: Prairie, farmland, a ravine, scenic views of the Capitol	**WHEELCHAIR ACCESSIBILITY:** Around scenic parking area and possibly some grassy trails
EXPOSURE: Mostly sun	
TRAFFIC: Light	**FACILITIES:** Portable toilets, water, picnic tables
TRAIL SURFACE: Mowed grass, some dirt, and cedar chip	**CONTACT:** popefarmconservancy.org
HIKING TIME: 1–1.5 hours	**COMMENTS:** No dogs allowed. The park is a work in progress, and trails will adapt to the needs of the park and crops, so the map may vary from time to time.
DRIVING DISTANCE: 2.2 miles west of the Beltline Highway (US 12/14) and Old Sauk Road exit	

Recessional moraines are rock and soil deposits left where the glacier paused as it receded, and there are two of them here. You are standing on the first; signage challenges you to find the second.

To your left is an opening in the stone fence. Cross here to the other side to find the wide mowed trails arranged in geometric order over the fields. You have options to go back and forth across the field between the various plantations. Go left, back along the stone wall, with a field of sunflowers to your right as the trail takes you downhill to two small gardens. The plants here exemplify the crops of the American Indians and the early pioneers. Just before them, the trail goes right, with the sunflowers on your right and a farm fence to your left. Only 500 feet later, the path goes to the right up the hill. (Future development may open up this trail to go straight here, with the ridge to the right and continuing west to the agricultural fields of the western side of the park.) At the crest of the hill, find oak savanna at the left. A trail goes right back toward the stone fence or follows left along the top of the hill, keeping the savanna on your left. There is a gate just past here on your left. This trail goes down through the oak savanna and follows the lower edge of the hill, heading west with oaks above you to the right. This area is sometimes closed.

If you skip the gate and go along the top of the ridge, you come to a circle of stones. The trail bends right, then brings you to another juncture. Right leads you back to the fence again. Go left alongside grain crops and down the hill, with that oak savanna still off to the left.

At the bottom of the hill, go left. Right is a cutoff trail skipping the western fields of the park. As you head left, take your first right as the trail goes along the north edge of an oak-covered hill. (Going straight brings you to that trail through the savanna beyond the gate you passed.) The trail ascends to a flattened top and offers a nice view of the neighboring farm. You can also see the oak savanna trail where it rejoins the fields and follows up the hill along the southern limit of the park and parallel to the path you are on. A path from your perch on this hill doubles back to it.

Pope Farm Park

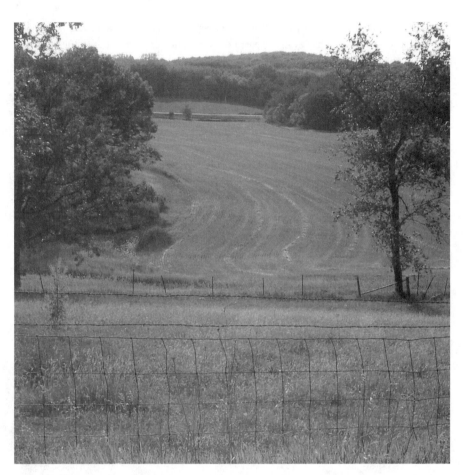

Views of farmland

Head west, following the trail toward Twin Valley Road. To the left is a little country church and more crops just outside the park. You can expect deer here in the early morning or toward dusk especially. Across the field to the right is mixed forest along the return trail, and you have a bit of altitude on the field to see it all.

Walk the 0.2 mile to the end of the field at the edge of the road. To the left, a trail takes you to a pedestrian entrance from Twin Valley Road. Go right along the road to the opposite side, where there's another map board. Go right again with the woods, at your left, populated by young black walnuts and long-needled pines and occasional oaks.

Keep along the edge of the woods as the trail goes left with the property line, where another juncture also offers you a path to the right that would take you back to where you've been. There's a map board here. You are now coming back into the middle section of the park; from the map board, it is another 750 feet to the next trail to the left. Keep along the edge of the woods until there.

The path left goes into the woods along a deep gully heading north with cedar-chip trail on either side of it. The cut in the earth is a dramatic contrast to the rolling hills, but before you head into the shade, continue forward on the trail less than 200 feet to see a bit of regional history.

On your left will be a spillway constructed by the Civilian Conservation Corps and used to capture the force of runoff. The rainwater enters the spillway and gathers in a basin before being released into the gorge, reducing its speed and preventing excessive erosion.

Backtrack to the trail into the woods. This footpath descends through predominantly locust, cottonwood, and oak. Along the right is a deep gully. Be careful of the trail edge, especially when cedar chips are fresh and give a false sense of stability. It's only 800 feet to the road, where you cross the bottom of the gully and climb back up to the other side to follow the trail back through the woods toward the spillway.

When you come out of the trees, go left, which is due east. If you haven't guessed already, this is the second moraine. You'll reach another small stone amphitheater that overlooks the Black Earth Creek valley and a ski jump in the distance.

Continuing east here, you have choices. Left takes you to the parking area along Blackhawk Road; right goes back to the stone fence and ultimately to where you started. Going straight is part of the Country Walk Trail and takes you through more crops along the edge of the eastern section of the park, which really does have the feel of a country road, minus the traffic and perhaps the dust. You are 0.4 mile from the parking lot if you go right. The trail before you will loop around 0.5 mile to the southern end of the lot.

Go straight where the prairie is loaded with wildflowers: coneflowers, bergamot, black-eyed Susans, sunflowers, and many others. A short distance along, the trail turns right (south), with prairie to your right and farm fields on the left, and then angles down to the southwest until it reaches the parking area.

Nearby Activities

For a great local Friday fish fry (or home-style cooking any other day), check out The Village Green at 7508 Hubbard Ave. in Middleton (608-831-9962).

GPS COORDINATES AND DIRECTIONS

N43° 04' 30.88" W89° 33' 58.12"

Exit the Beltline Highway (US 12/14) at Old Sauk Road and go 2.2 miles west. The park entrance is on the right. Park in the first parking lot on your left. The trailhead is at the northwest corner of the lot.

16 Tenney Park to Schenk's Corners

The lagoon at Tenney Park

In Brief

Follow the Yahara River from the locks at Lake Mendota to its outlet into Lake Monona, and then stop in for a drink or a bite to eat in one of Madison's long-standing neighborhoods.

Description

From the parking lot, cross Sherman Avenue to the corner of Marston Avenue. Follow the asphalt path to the left as it passes through some trees. Halfway down the block, the trail goes right and crosses a 1929 stone bridge over the Tenney Park lagoon. It is photogenic any time of the year, but especially when the lily pads are out. On the other side is a bench where the path continues through the park. The first trail juncture leads left over another bridge to a parking lot, but stay right. At the next juncture, another trail goes right to

LENGTH & CONFIGURATION: 3.9-mile misshapen lollipop	**ACCESS:** Park portions are open 5 a.m.–10 p.m.
DIFFICULTY: Easy	**MAPS:** USGS *Madison East;* **visitmadison.com**
SCENERY: Two lakes, river, locks, residential neighborhoods	
	WHEELCHAIR ACCESSIBILITY: Yes
EXPOSURE: Mixed	**FACILITIES:** Restrooms, water, picnic areas, playgrounds, changing rooms, lighted tennis courts, boat landings at Tenney Park; several restaurants and bars in the Atwood-Schenk's Corners area
TRAFFIC: Moderate	
TRAIL SURFACE: Asphalt, concrete, some grass, and dirt	
HIKING TIME: 1.5–2 hours	**CONTACT: visitmadison.com**
DRIVING DISTANCE: 1.7 miles from the Capitol Square	**COMMENTS:** No dogs allowed in Tenney Park

another bridge. Again stay straight, and the path takes you to a metal bridge over the water leading left, nearly on the other side of the block-long park.

At the end of the bridge, go left through the parking lot until you come to the Yahara Parkway Bike Path to the right as it goes south along the Yahara River. There is an observation platform at the water's edge. Facing south, you'll see a ramp going right up to Johnson Street; stay on the trail and follow it through the short tunnel under the street (this is lighted at night). On the other side, the trail resumes along the river; at 0.1 mile, you will cross railroad tracks. The rail bed is no longer operational and a metal bridge goes left over the water. The trail to the left is a spur that connects out to Johnson Street. Continue straight and at 0.1 mile pass under Washington Avenue (with exits up to the street and a bus stop for bus routes 6, 14, 15, 27, 29, 56, and 57). This is Steensland Bridge, named for a Norwegian consul and former Madison resident Halle Steensland. Originally built in 1904, it was replaced in 2006 with the current construction, which is in the Prairie School style of architecture. At night, it is well lit and quite attractive. The path beneath is very wide, but stay aware of bicyclists.

One block later, cross Main Street, and half a block later some railroad tracks. It's another half block to a cul-de-sac at Thornton Avenue and Williamson Street. The Capital City Trail crosses from left to right on an asphalt path. At the corner to your right is Mickey's Tavern (608-251-9964), which also serves good food and features live music.

Go left from the cul-de-sac on the Capital City Trail as it takes you across the Yahara River on an old metal railroad bridge. Come to traffic lights at Williamson Street. Cross here (there is a button to force the change of lights) and head down Riverside Drive on the sidewalk in a residential neighborhood to Jenifer Street. Cross the river back the other way on the pedestrian bridge, and go left down Thornton Avenue another block to Rutledge Street to a bench and some prairie flowers.

The mouth of the Yahara River where it empties into Lake Monona is just beyond, and you can find a picnic table and a small green space there, but nothing more. Cross the

Tenney Park to Schenk's Corners

The breakwater near the locks—an excellent place to watch the sun set

bridge at Rutledge Street. (You could have just stayed on Riverside Drive, of course, but I am a fan of crossing bridges.) On the other side, a dirt trail goes down to the right into Yahara Place Park. The footpath follows 0.4 mile of the shore of Lake Monona, with cottonwoods and willows for shade. There is a playground here, as well as picnic tables and rocks along the shore that make nice meditative perches. This is a wonderful spot in the morning when the sun is rising. Or find something to do along the hike for the rest of the day, and then come back, because the end of the trail is the perfect spot for a sunset.

At the end of the park, come to Dunning Street. Take this left five blocks (0.3 mile) to Atwood Avenue. At the corner on the right is the Harmony Bar, which has excellent pizza. The recipe for the dough is akin to a state secret.

Cross the busy Atwood Avenue and go left. This is the Atwood-Schenk's Corners neighborhood. Coming up on your left is Monty's Blue Plate Diner, a Madison classic for breakfast. On your right is the Barrymore Theatre. Built in 1929 as the Eastwood, it was the third movie theater in Madison. Today it brings in nearly 100 live music concerts each year.

There are various small restaurants along this four-block stretch, and the neighborhood hosts a festival every July. You will come to Schenk's Corners where Atwood meets Winnebago Street. The building at 2009 Winnebago Street was formerly Schenk General Store, which sold everything from groceries and housewares to cigars and clothing. Alchemy Café, right across the street, has a good fish fry on Fridays and is a beer connoisseur's tavern. Tex Tubb's Taco Palace and One Barrel Brewing also sit along this famous intersection.

Cross Winnebago at the traffic light and go left on the other side, passing before the bank building there and following Winnebago Street back to Williamson Street to the traffic lights to pick up the Capital City Trail once again. Go back over the bridge and retrace your steps along the Yahara River to Tenney Park.

When you come back through the tunnel under Johnson Street, follow the asphalt path along the park road straight out to Sherman Avenue and cross the street to the entry road to the locks. If you go right across the bridge on Sherman Avenue, there is a boat landing on the north side of the street. Just above it to the east (right) are several park benches perfect for a chat or sunset viewing. You can also watch boats pass through the locks from the bridge.

The hike continues across Sherman Avenue, passing the locks office where you can find water, restrooms, and a picnic table. There is a wheelchair-accessible ramp to a fishing platform. Originally, there was an earthen dam on this spot, where a gristmill, sawmill, and brewery operated. Locks were built to replace it in 1896. These were replaced in 1959. The water level in Lake Mendota is 5 feet higher than that of Lake Monona.

Go around the lock building to the left and find the breakwater. You can follow this out to its point. Rocks line the concrete sidewalk, and benches are spaced out evenly along its length. The view of the Capitol and the university is perfect, and the sun sets over the lake from here.

Coming back from the point, go right (west) along the shore of Lake Mendota, and a crushed-rock trail takes you past the small beach area to the parking lot. A massive willow split down the middle still grows in all directions on a small point to your right and offers another fine place to take a break. There are restrooms in the changing house, and there's a drinking fountain at the entrance to the lot. Bus routes 2 and 27 stop here.

Nearby Activities

This side of town is neighborhood-proud. Yahara Place Park is the site of Marquette Neighborhood Waterfront Festival in June. Atwoodfest and Schenk's Corners neighborhood festivals are in July and August, respectively. Just west of this hike are La Fete de Marquette around July 14, the Orton Park Festival in August, and the Willy Street Festival in September. Check **madison.com** for an events calendar. Also be sure to visit the lovely Olbrich Botanical Gardens (**olbrich.org**) farther east at 3330 Atwood Ave.

GPS COORDINATES AND DIRECTIONS
N43° 05' 33.72" W89° 22' 19.91"

From the Capitol Square, go east on East Washington 1.2 miles to Baldwin Street. Go left 0.5 mile to Sherman Avenue and turn right. The parking lot is on your left one block later. The trailhead begins at the parking lot entrance.

17 Token Creek

A boardwalk follows Token Creek.

In Brief

Follow a trail and boardwalk along a clear country creek, explore sedge meadow and prairie, and finish the day with a round of disc golf.

Description

At the end of the last Ice Age, drainage of this area was blocked, and the soggy land supported plant life that, as it died and decayed, became the alkaline peat deposits now beneath the marsh. In the 1930s, dredging lowered the water level, allowing prairie to invade. Sedges lost out to lavender asters, sunflowers, and goldenrods, which bloom in late summer. Token Creek and some wetlands remain, but prairie closes in around them as the creek makes its meager way to the Yahara River via the northern reaches of Cherokee Marsh to the west.

From the park gate, continue to Shelter #2 just past the campgrounds. Find a map board at the trailhead across from the shelter. A map box to the left should have trail maps, or you can go to one of the campsite hosts and ask for one.

LENGTH & CONFIGURATION: 3.7-mile loop	**MAPS:** USGS *De Forest;* available at trailhead or from campsite manager
DIFFICULTY: Easy	**WHEELCHAIR ACCESSIBILITY:** Yes, on boardwalk and most grassy trails in dry conditions
SCENERY: Prairie, marsh, flowing water, and some mixed woods	
EXPOSURE: Only partly shaded	**FACILITIES:** Restrooms, campsites, playgrounds, disc-golf course, vending machine, bridle areas, and shelters
TRAFFIC: Light	
TRAIL SURFACE: Mowed paths, some packed dirt, and a boardwalk	**CONTACT: countyofdane.com/lwrd/ parks/token_creek.aspx**
HIKING TIME: 1.5 hours	**COMMENTS:** Dogs are allowed leashed or unleashed in fee-controlled dog areas. The fee is $5 daily and $30 annually. A smaller fenced area is reserved for small dogs. Horses share some trails with hikers and always have the right-of-way. Disc golfers pay an $8 daily fee for using the course.
DRIVING DISTANCE: 0.5 mile north on US 51 from the I-39 juncture	
ACCESS: Year-round 5 a.m.–10 p.m. except for campers	

Starting from the trail board, follow along the road to the tall grass. A cross-country ski trail starts here and follows the road deeper into the park, but go right toward the creek edge to pick up another trail. Go left, with the creek on your right, following a mowed path. This takes you through tall grasses and some willows before the trail turns left and connects to that original cross-country trail. Go right and find a trail marker for Trails 1, 2, and 3. Follow along the edge of the park road. You can see the highway intersection from this clearing, and, through this first portion of the park, you will have traffic noise and the occasional plane passing overhead from the nearby Dane County airport. The trail is open to the sun for 900 feet, and then you pass into woods. There's a spur trail to the left to the road. After this juncture, the hiking trail joins the horse trail. It is mostly shaded by a mix of maple, oak, and black walnut.

Come back out to the road and a gate. The trail is really the grassy shoulder of the road. Stay right alongside it and pass between two wooden posts. Pass a roadside parking area, after which the trail goes right back into oak forest and slopes down. Follow it as it curves right gently down the hill through oaks. Look for a few young shagbark hickories through here. The forest is bustling with chipmunks, squirrels, and stirrings in the undergrowth as the trail dips at some cedar chips. At a yield sign at a trail juncture, go left and reemerge into the sun. This is the closest to the highway that you will be, and highway noise can be quite loud here.

Pass behind the third hole of the disc golf course and find the end of Trail 1 at this juncture. Continue straight on Trail 2 and 3. You are partly shaded by pine as you walk along, with the fairway to your left on the other side of the line of trees. The trail bends to the right and back with a gentle S, and the air is redolent with long-needle pines. As you pass a clump of sumac, the pines become taller and you pass a trail sign as the trail

Token Creek

turns left just inside the boundaries of the park. You can see residences to the right through the trees.

To the left is grassy meadow with a few trees starting to take hold. From this point, traffic noise fades significantly, and there is a bench in the shade to the right where you can sit and watch birds active in the prairie. Just past this, find another trail marker as the trail bends right through a short corridor of sumac before crossing the field to the end of the park road and a turnaround there. Trails to the left just before this are part of the bridle trails and an exercise circle for the horses.

Cross the turnaround and enter the woods again on the other side. There's an entry trail to the park from the right 400 feet from here, where the main trail goes left along the western boundary of the dog exercise area. There is parking along Anderson Road just outside the gate. Continue to the left on the mostly shaded trail of cedar chips that soon give way to grass and packed dirt. The trail bends left and brings you to another trail marker at the entrance to the pet exercise area to your right. Pass the entrance and follow the cut path with trail markers 2 and 3.

Stay straight on Trail 3. The left path is Trail 2, which eventually loops out and back through the meadow to your left through the disc golf fairways to rejoin this trail again. Pass a spur trail on the right to a private gate, and then, as you reach the other side of the open field, the return trail for Trail 2 is on your left. Soon after, you come to another fork in the road. Go right here for a short loop with no horse access that curves out and back a bit farther up the trail. Go right at the trail marker when you return to the main. Just past here is a cutoff trail that leads back to the parking lot. Stay to the right instead and head out into open meadow again. At the other side, come to the Trail 2 juncture that goes left toward the parking lots. Go straight on Trail 3. Look for an old red barn with a rooster weathervane through the trees outside the park to the right. On the other side of the field, another trail heads left to a bench. Go straight and check out the enormous aspens with massive trunks to your left. To your right just outside the park, see another park with playgrounds. A couple of unofficial trails cross 30 feet of tall grass to get there.

You are now walking along a ditch with some standing water to your left. Cross a creek with wooden railings. Prairie awaits you at the end of the brush line; look for a tall dead tree next to a low area with standing water and algae on your left. Watch for some sandpipers and perhaps cranes or herons. Swallows skim the tops of the grasses. Duck back into thick woods on a packed-earth trail often showing tracks of deer and other animals. The shade lasts another 600 feet, and you have to cross a low muddy area about 6 feet across with a culvert in the middle before crossing another meadow.

At the other side of a bridge, the trail crosses a tiny creek and the path returns to shade. Now you can see Token Creek to the right before crossing another bridge. Look for lilies along the water's edge. The trail ventures left into a campsite. Go around the site unless it is unoccupied; the trail picks up on the other side, where a strip of old asphalt heads back into the tall grass. Pass under some trees to find the beginning of the boardwalk. It goes left at a right angle and passes through a swampy area with an abundance of willows as it follows Token Creek curving right. This is the nicest part of the trail, easy to walk, secluded, and putting you right along the waterway through brush and sedge meadow. A boardwalk spur goes left to the wheelchair-accessible campsite. Stay straight and cross a bridge over another small creek feeding into the bigger Token Creek. Willows provide some shade up to the end of the boardwalk at the park road. Educational signage here gives information about the 0.5-mile boardwalk segment of the trail and touts the springtime sky dance of woodcocks, which can be seen in open areas of the meadow.

You have the option of following the park road back to the parking lot. Otherwise, go right to the park entrance gate, where there is an observation platform across the road overlooking a wide area of the creek. This segment of the trail is also a dog exercise area. The trail continues to follow the creek, and cedar trees start to appear. Come to a gate on your left and a trail to the right over a culvert (which may suffer from erosion and wash-outs) onto a small island in the stream. It's a short loop around and back, and you can find a "sacred circle" built by friends of the park where cedars surround a small boulder. Black-birds pay close attention to you in late spring when they nest around here. On the opposite side of the island, take the fork to the left; the right trail is a short dead end, but you can climb out onto the rocks in the stream from there.

Go right back on the main trail and pass a small spur that merely goes through the grass to the water's edge. Just past here, find a volleyball court to the left, but keep right, continuing along the creek, visible now through the weeds to the right. The next intersection is another island loop. Go right over a concrete bridge with a culvert that allows this narrow branch of the creek to pass. Cross onto a second larger island. The trail follows the perimeter, offering some looks into the water and a couple of maple-shaded spots in an otherwise sunny meadow.

Returning to the concrete bridge, cross back to the main trail, go right, and then take the branch to the left to get to your car, which should already be visible from here.

Winter is nice for hikes along the boardwalk and nearby portions of the trails, where you can easily find animal tracks—and the woodcocks' springtime sky dance is not something you see just anywhere.

Nearby Activities

Pine Cone Restaurant (608-249-8778) right outside the park is a truck stop and greasy spoon with cheap eats and coffee—nothing fancy, just hearty highway fare.

GPS COORDINATES AND DIRECTIONS
N43° 10' 57.05" W89° 19' 9.64"

Take US 51 north out of Madison until you pass under the I-39 interchange. Almost a half mile north of here, find Token Creek Lane, just past a truck stop on the right. Turn here and follow the lane to the park entrance gate. From the gate, follow the park road 0.25 mile and park on the right side near the trail board.

18 Tom George Greenway

The trailhead at Cottage Grove Road

In Brief

This chain of three small neighborhood parks is more of a secret garden. The narrow stretch of green space on either side of Cottage Grove Road is a nice short hike that begs you to linger amid oaks and wildflowers.

Description

This place seems like a well-kept secret, and here I am blowing its cover. The hike actually traverses three separate parks, but you wouldn't know it. Elvehjem Sanctuary to the south was named for Conrad A. Elvehjem. Born in nearby McFarland, he was a renowned UW professor and biochemist who first identified and discovered the importance of the vitamin niacin. Heritage Prairie Conservation Park to the north is another neighborhood park featuring a prairie remnant on a rocky hill. Tom George Greenway, named for a

LENGTH & CONFIGURATION: 2.2-mile double out-and-back	**ACCESS:** 4 a.m.–1 hour after sunset
DIFFICULTY: Easy to moderate	**MAPS:** USGS *Madison East*
SCENERY: Mixed forest, highway overlook, prairie	**WHEELCHAIR ACCESSIBILITY:** None
EXPOSURE: Mostly shaded	**FACILITIES:** None on the trail, but Elvehjem Park has a shelter and restrooms
TRAFFIC: Light	
TRAIL SURFACE: Packed dirt	**CONTACT:** See Elvehjem Park or Heritage Prairie at **cityofmadison.com/ parks/parks**
HIKING TIME: 1 hour	
DRIVING DISTANCE: 1 mile east of US 51 on County Road BB	**COMMENTS:** No dogs allowed

former alderperson who used a lot of his own funds to beautify the Cottage Grove Boulevard, connects the two parks with a trail.

This can all be a little confusing, depending on the entrance you take. I recommend the trailhead on the north side of Cottage Grove Road and then doing two out-and-backs from this central point. Alternative entrances can be found at Heritage Prairie on Queensbridge Road or the Elvehjem Sanctuary on Academy Road at the south end.

A grassy trail descends off the edge of the sidewalk where you'd hardly suspect to find a hiking trail. Mixed forest surrounds you, and tall grass stands along the intermittent water to your left where a concrete storm-runoff culvert emerges from under Cottage Grove Road. Large rocks have been placed here to stop erosion at the opening. Residences are just a stone's throw to either side of this corridor of green space, and 300 feet in, the path becomes packed dirt. Expect songbirds, butterflies, and wildflowers throughout the park, and the occasional coyote scat is evidence of bigger visitors. At the opposite side of the first small clearing, cross a culvert and follow the trail back into woods.

Brush closes in around you. Highway noise from I-94 rises in the distance. Soon the terrain to your left slopes up a bit, and tall cottonwoods fill out the canopy. The trail widens as you pass a storm drain to your right. Cross over another culvert and through some more trees before the trail opens to the sky with tall grass on either side and pines lining the path. A trail leads up to the right through sumac, a potential cutoff for your return path. Keep going past this to a fork in the trail. Left will take you across the ditch to your left and out of the park to Queensbridge Road, where a sign marks the trail as the entry to Heritage Prairie Conservation Park. This is an alternative starting point with on-street parking. The path to the right splits as well. The right branch is your return path, and the left trail goes into the woods where the canopy reaches over you but doesn't quite block out the sky. This trail goes up the hill, becoming crushed stone in a few places. At the top you find medium-size oaks, and then the trail curves to the right. Beyond the brush to your left is the highway.

Come to another fork in the trail with a metal fence post to the right. To the left is a spur trail that leads to an opening in the park fence and a view of the highway and the

Tom George Greenway

Butterflies and wildflowers are common along the trail.

Cottage Grove Road police station. The trail to the right goes down the hill, steeply passing through bushes as it makes its way back to where you started the climb up the hill. The aforementioned cutoff trail is to your left as you descend, and you can opt for that, which is a bit steeper. At the bottom, you can retrace your steps to Cottage Grove Road for the second half of this hike.

However, there is more to explore here if you are willing—though the trail isn't always clear. If you go to the left-leading path toward the park exit on Queensbridge Road, you might see a faint trail through the grass that follows along the right side of the ditch heading toward the highway. This follows a wider loop of about 0.2 mile up that hill to your right. As you follow the shrinking ditch on your left, watch for a much clearer path about 300 feet from the juncture. This will lead to the right up the hill through a clump of aspens as you approach the curve at the top. The trail goes up a bit more and widens out. To your right, the earth drops away into a small gully with some exposed rocks in the understory. The highway is again to your left, and you are on the outside of the fence at the crest of the grassy ridge. Go to the right along the fence to find that gate that leads you back into the park and follows the return path down the hill once again.

Retrace your steps to Cottage Grove Road. Cross the street to the south side and enter the woods there on the western side of the storm sewer. Once again, the trail quickly draws you from a well-manicured residential neighborhood and a busy street into an unexpected tangle of woods.

Now you are heading south, and it is quieter without I-94 nearby. Spur trails to either side lead to backyards. The trail surface shows more tree roots and is more rugged. The character of the terrain is different. You will see more basswoods and some black walnuts as well as red oaks. This side seems more like a ravine and a thicker forest. The area is suitable for tree houses and children's forts (you may find one), and with more fallen wood, fungi hunters will have more to see than wildflower fans. The canopy is thick.

Come to an intersection where the trail to the left heads uphill and exits the park on the sidewalk on Painted Post Drive, with crushed rock about halfway up. Stay right. Sandy patches appear in the trail. The trail rises moderately through dirt, sand, tree roots, and some dead-leaf cover, and then passes around a giant oak tree. Watch for a trail to the left up to an elementary school where there are picnic tables in a mowed park. Other little footpaths lead right to more backyards.

Come to a T-intersection. The left trail heads up to that school; go right down the hill a bit until the main trail bends left again so that it continues through the middle of the forest. Come to a large rock that marks a trail to a conical mound. The mound was constructed by a hunting and gathering culture around 400 A.D. and was used to mark where they met to bury their dead. You can follow this spur trail right just 20 feet, but there is little sign of the mound itself.

Continuing along the main path, pass a post to the right that reads ELVEHJEM SANCTUARY CONSERVATION PARK. One hundred feet after this, the trail enters a mowed park area with a ball diamond and Elvehjem Elementary School to the left. The trail sign is set back into the woods and not easily seen if you choose to start your hike from this park on Academy Drive to the west of the school. Elvehjem Park has a shelter and restrooms. Retrace your steps back to Cottage Grove Road, or you can walk east toward the school to pick up Ellen Avenue and follow it north to Cottage Grove Road.

Nearby Activities

Stop in at Culver's for the custard of the day or a famous "butter burger" on Cottage Grove Road just before you return to US 51 (Stoughton Road). In mid-May, nearby Heritage Sanctuary, at 600 Meadowlark Drive, is awash with trilliums and a short walk from the entrance to Heritage Prairie.

GPS COORDINATES AND DIRECTIONS

N43° 05' 4.42" W89° 17' 30.37"

From US 51 (Stoughton Road), take CR BB (Cottage Grove Road) east 1 mile. Parking is on the street at the trailhead near a large wooden sign that says TOM GEORGE GREENWAY. Park on the westbound side of the street. The trailhead is 70 feet to the right of the sign.

NORTHWEST

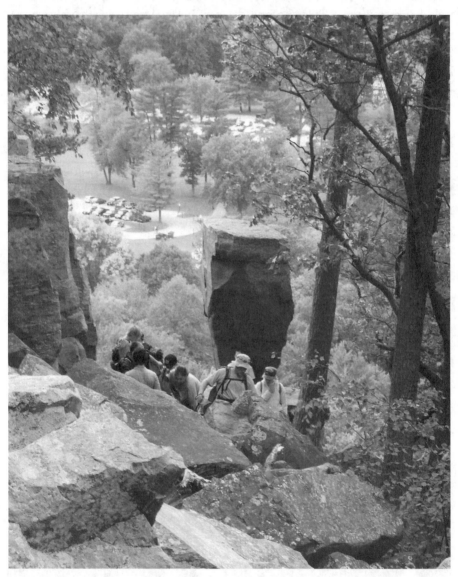

Ice Age Trail: Devil's Lake Segment (see page 130)

19 Black Hawk Unit: Lower Wisconsin State Riverway

In Brief

Look out over the Wisconsin River valley from several scenic overlooks as you hike through restored prairies and rich forests with ravines. This is the land where warrior Black Hawk once turned to face the pursuing U.S. Army and militia to buy his people time to escape across the river.

Description

The woods are thick, the prairies are full of flowers, and the overlooks show the hilly landscape of the Wisconsin River valley. A spot so beautiful also witnessed a sad bit of history. Black Hawk, a Sauk warrior, led 60 warriors against 700 militia at the Battle of Wisconsin Heights. The bold maneuver—perhaps the only time Black Hawk's band turned around to face the pursuers—was costly to the Indians but bought time for nearly 1,000

LENGTH & CONFIGURATION: 9.5-mile double loop	**DRIVING DISTANCE:** 19.7 miles north from US 14/University Avenue and US 12
DIFFICULTY: Easy, moderate, and difficult sections	**ACCESS:** 6 a.m.–11 p.m.
SCENERY: Mixed forest, prairie, scenic overlooks, effigy mounds	**MAPS:** USGS *Black Earth;* on map boards at trail junctures and parking lot
EXPOSURE: Mostly shaded with open prairie sections	**WHEELCHAIR ACCESSIBILITY:** None
TRAFFIC: Light	**FACILITIES:** Portable toilets, shelters, water
TRAIL SURFACE: Mowed grass, packed dirt, sandy patches, some crushed stone	**CONTACT: lwr.state.wi.us**
HIKING TIME: 4 hours	**COMMENTS:** Mosquitoes can be harsh here. Leashed dogs allowed except when trails are groomed for skiing.

women, children, and elderly people to cross the Wisconsin River and escape. The success was short-lived, as many were soon slaughtered or drowned at the Battle of Bad Axe trying to escape across the Mississippi River.

Start up Wachter Road at the special events entryway. The gate is typically closed, and there is a map board next to it. At 0.15 mile, go left on a packed-dirt and sand footpath into the forest for 0.1 mile, where you will come to a trail juncture. The hike described here divides the park into two halves. Go right for the first giant loop, and then return to this spot to go left for the second loop.

The right path heads 0.3 mile uphill on sandy terrain with pine forest to the left. After the easy pass along the pines, the trail is at its roughest, with tree roots, sandy patches, and loose sandstone at a moderate incline. At times the surrounding plants reach into the trail and grab at you as you pass. At 0.3 mile, a spur trail goes left into the brush off the official map. It is difficult to see, is not maintained, and follows the top of the ridge, where it peters out about 0.1 mile into the woods.

Two hundred feet past the spur is an intersection. To the left is private land; go right 0.2 mile, still on dirt and broken rock and a bit steep until you come to a T. Go left on a wide dirt and grass trail. At 0.1 mile, the trail rounds a point where a ski trail parts to the right at a map board. Continue straight as the trail curves back around, heading south 0.2 mile to another spur trail left. Continue another 300 feet to a clearing. Go straight, as a little lollipop trail takes you to what is a scenic overlook when foliage is thin or absent. A sign says as much: TRAIL ENDS AT OVERLOOK. You'll return to this clearing and stay to the leftmost (when returning) path leading out and downhill 0.15 mile to the next juncture, with a cutoff trail to the right into the open. There is a map board there as well. Go left and continue down, with nice views to the left.

Another 0.25 mile brings you to the edge of some prairie and a trail that heads to the right over the hill and to the center of the park. Continue straight along the edge of the trees and pass through more woods downhill, round a corner, and come to a small pond

Dew collecting on some berries

with bullfrogs and cattails. From the pond, the trail goes left into the woods for a 0.4-mile segment that runs up and down along a ravine, briefly passing through open canopy but otherwise shaded. From there, head into prairie, passing 0.15 mile through wildflowers to the other end of that prairie cutoff trail you passed earlier at the other end. There's a map here and a straight path that is a ski trail coming down from the hill with the overlook lollipop. Go to the right into the prairie toward a clump of bushes to get the scenic overlook from the top of the hill. Look for the hills of Baraboo and the Wisconsin River valley to the northwest. Double back to the park center, and pass a horse pavilion on the left and a boardwalk to the right to another pavilion.

There is a water pump here and portable toilets near a log cabin. Hike past the cabin to the park road. You'll see that the road heads right and passes a barn off to your right. But go left on mowed paths into prairie. One hundred feet along on your right is your return path to this spot. Go straight another 200 feet to a trail map and juncture of three trails. Go left through prairie surrounded by forest. These paths are easier than the forest trails, with more level surfaces and less of an incline. It's 0.7 mile down this trail to the next juncture. Pass a pond on the left as you come around the back end of the field. There's a nice panorama of the area around you. The path follows the edge of the prairie and heads into trees. At the juncture, go left to follow a 0.8-mile finger loop into the woods. You can also go right here to skip this and the next two similar loops into the forest and head back through prairie to the park center.

When you finish the finger loop, go left at the next juncture to hike the next 0.3-mile loop. A trail to the right allows you to skip it and brings you to that same prairie path that heads east (right) to the park center. At the juncture at the end of this second finger loop is a four-way intersection. To the right is that prairie path cutoff coming at you. Straight continues the larger park loop but cuts off the next 0.4-mile loop to the left, if you prefer. Otherwise, go left on that third loop and come to a trail at 0.15 mile that goes left and long out of the park to another park entry. Stay right, and the trail curves right and back, passing a spur trail on the left and continuing to the next juncture, which is the loop's cutoff path on the right. Go left instead, keeping the pines to your right. There's a scenic overlook on the left at 0.1 mile with two benches on either side of a little clearing. Past here it is 0.6 mile back to the park center if you take the next juncture to the left. (Going right at that juncture cuts that distance to 0.3 mile.)

Follow the park road past the storage barn 0.7 mile down the hill back to where you first entered the woods near the trailhead (on the right now). Go back into the woods, this time bearing left at the first intersection. This sandy path will take you north 0.1 mile to a juncture. Left goes to another parking lot on WI 78 and is also your return path for this loop. Go straight 0.5 mile on a rolling, grassy trail mostly shaded by thick hardwood forest. Look for some exposed rock above you to the right and wildflowers along the path. You reach a juncture where a trail to the right goes out and back 0.1 mile each way to a collection of American Indian effigy mounds.

Returning to this juncture from the mounds, go right (east) another 0.1 mile, pass a trail bearing left, and find a 0.15-mile out-and-back trail on the right steeply climbing to what is an overlook when foliage is down. From the bottom of that spur trail, head east (right) another 0.1 mile, crossing a bridge to get to a T juncture. Go right here and take a 0.5-mile turn through brush and then up a ridge to another short spur-trail overlook on the left side of the trail before descending again to the other end of the cutoff trail to your left. The cutoff skips the climb and reduces the distance by 0.4 mile.

From that juncture after your trek over the hill, go to the right, passing a right-bound exit trail to private property and coming 0.1 mile to another juncture. Go right toward the edge of the park along the highway. Another trail goes right to private property; head left along the road 400 feet to a historical marker and wayside. Keep following the trail into the woods running parallel to the highway. Another 0.4 mile takes you to the second parking lot. The trail continues into the woods at the other end 0.15 mile to a juncture you already passed to start this loop. Go right back to Wachter Road, and then go right again down that park road to the original parking lot.

Nearby Activities

Serving deli sandwiches, salads, ice cream, and coffee, and offering a patio overlooking the Wisconsin River, the Blue Spoon Café is a nice place to stop after your hike (550 Water St., Prairie du Sac; 608-643-0837; **bluespooncafe.com**).

20 Devil's Lake State Park: East Bluff

The view of the north shore from the east bluff

In Brief

Forget the StairMaster—this is a natural workout with a view. Climb to the top of a towering bluff overlooking Devil's Lake, and then explore the woods and prairie beyond.

Description

The hike starts with Balanced Rock Trail, which zigzags up the broken rock of the bluff face. In just about 0.3 mile, you climb nearly 500 feet from the base of the bluff to the scenic overlook. The trail heads into the woods between the bluff and the parking lot, and you cross over railroad tracks and follow a packed dirt trail to where the broken rock marks the bottom of the bluff. The trail is clearly marked and steps have been fashioned using the stones and patches of asphalt along the way. You pass Balanced Rock at about 0.2 mile.

At the top of the climb is a wonderful overlook to the right from a large flat area of stone. Turkey vultures ride the thermals here. Go left to find a trail intersection with a map and an emergency box to the left. A trail to the left is your return path; the one to the right along the cliff is part of the Ice Age Trail: Devil's Lake Segment. Go straight from the cliff into the woods on the East Bluff Woods Trail. You'll be going downhill for a long way now.

LENGTH & CONFIGURATION: 5.6-mile loop

DIFFICULTY: Difficult

SCENERY: Cliffs, lake overlook, mixed forest

EXPOSURE: Exposed on the steep climb, otherwise mostly shaded

TRAFFIC: Moderate at the cliffs, light in the forest

TRAIL SURFACE: Stepping-stones, asphalt, crushed rock

HIKING TIME: 2–2.5 hours

DRIVING DISTANCE: 33.2 miles from US 12 and University Avenue

ACCESS: 6 a.m.–11 p.m. year-round

MAPS: USGS *Baraboo;* online at **dnr. state.wi.us;** at park office

WHEELCHAIR ACCESSIBILITY: None

FACILITIES: Restrooms, campgrounds, water, changing rooms at the beach

CONTACT: dnr.wi.gov/topic/parks/ name/devilslake, 608-356-8301

COMMENTS: Devil's Lake requires some care and common sense. Several people have fallen to their deaths from the cliffs. Stay on trails and do not climb. Leashed dogs allowed. All vehicles require a park sticker ($7 daily, $25 annual for vehicles with WI plates). Devil's Lake State Park is part of the Ice Age National Scientific Reserve, so vehicle fees are waived for holders of Federal passes. The park participates in the Junior Ranger/Wisconsin Explorer program (see Preface, page 8).

Start into mixed forest with blue sky beyond the edge of the woods to your right. At 0.15 mile, at the first intersection to the left, is East Bluff Woods Trail. Go right on a two-tire path. Follow this 0.3 mile, passing a trail to the right to Devil's Doorway at 0.1 mile and to The Potholes at 0.15 mile. These are geological features worth exploring: a sort of gateway of stone and depressions in the stone caused by erosion from rocks swirling in the eddies of flowing glacial meltwater.

At 0.3 mile, the trail leaves the access road and goes right at a large #5 sign. Pass a path to Moldy Buttress, a climbing point at 0.2 mile on the right, and D'Arcy's Buttress just about 0.1 mile after that. Continue as the trail starts to descend a bit and curves left on crushed stone with occasional eroded areas until you reach a trail juncture 0.2 mile later.

There is a bench to the right. The straight trail is the Uplands Trail, but left is your course, which is East Bluff Woods Trail *and* Uplands Trail. Follow this 0.25 mile downhill, and then notice a ditch joins it on the left. You then arrive at a trail marker, intersection, and bench. To the left is just the access road to the top of the bluff. East Bluff and Uplands trails become one as you continue straight 0.2 mile until you see a trail to the right. This is the East Bluff Woods Trail and the Steinke Basin Loop. Follow it and immediately come to a T. The right branch loops south and then north to the Ice Age Trail before coming back west to make the loop. Go left here and pass through a low-lying area with a bit of prairie with lilies and other wildflowers. Cross a small footbridge over an intermittent creek and pass a bench on the left. The unshaded grassy trail runs 0.25 mile from the T intersection to a second bridge in a clearing and then 0.1 mile to the intersection of the Uplands Trail. Go straight across on Steinke Basin/East Bluff Woods Trail.

The next 0.4 mile is through aspen colonies with some slender maples and hickories fighting for canopy dominance. At the next juncture, find Johnson Moraine Loop/Uplands Trail/Steinke Basin Trail to the right. Go left on East Bluff Woods Trail through scattered deadwood and rock. From here, it's 0.7 mile to a bridge, and there is sunlight just after that at the park's amphitheater. Along the way, however, watch for spur trails to the left out over tree roots to a drop-off of 20–35 feet that creates a sort of canyon area behind the much larger lakeside bluff.

At the amphitheater, an asphalt trail cuts behind it. Cross to a trail that goes back into the woods. Another 0.1 mile takes you to the park road. Go left and follow the serpentine road 0.25 mile all the way down to the parking lot, always staying left. Into the parking lot, follow along the left edge to find this lot's own trailhead with a kiosk and toilets.

Follow the crushed-stone path 0.1 mile into the woods to the first juncture with a map board and a place to clean off your boots. Take the East Bluff Trail to the right on rough asphalt through a cathedral of towering trees as it climbs once again to the top of the bluff and follows its edge. To the left at the juncture is the East Bluff Woods Trail, which stays far from the cliffs but nevertheless will run parallel and take you to the Balanced Rock Trail and scenic overlook where you first came up.

The East Bluff Trail climb is not as steep as Balanced Rock, but it goes on a bit longer. It is 1 mile from the juncture to the head of the Balanced Rock Trail. The first 0.7-mile climb through the rocky outcroppings offers a variety of nooks and crannies and overlooks to explore. The asphalt trail makes it easy to follow, and some places show steps of stone and asphalt. At some points, it dips and rises again with the bluff, and in various places it goes farther into the woods before swinging out again toward the cliffs.

At 0.7 mile, there is a cutoff trail to East Bluff Woods Trail. Stay right to keep on level trail the next 0.3 mile to the lookout point and trail juncture at the head of Balanced Rock Trail. Go to the right and follow that back down to the trailhead.

Nearby Activities

Ski Hi Fruit Farm, at E11219A Ski-Hi Road in Baraboo, just west of the park, offers 30 types of apples, unpasteurized cider, and various other local products. Apple season is usually late August to November, at which time the farm is open seven days a week. Call 608-356-3695 for more information.

GPS COORDINATES AND DIRECTIONS
N43° 24' 43.09" W89° 43' 28.21"

From University Avenue in Middleton, go north on US 12 for 30 miles to Ski Hi Road. Go right 1.25 miles to South Shore Road and turn right again. Follow this road 1.6 miles as it curves left and enters the park, taking you 1.6 miles to the parking lot for the south shore of the lake. Pick up the asphalt walking path at the north end of the parking lot for the trailhead.

21 Devil's Lake State Park: West Bluff

The view from the west bluff to the east bluff

In Brief

No less impressive than its sister bluff across the lake, this rocky outcropping offers a stroll along the lakeshore through talus and a series of overlooks 500 feet above the water.

Description

Devil's Lake might be a river, if not for a glacier's intrusion about 15,000 years ago. The two bluffs seen today are two of the most ancient rock outcrops in North America. Estimated to be about 1.6 billion years old, they are made of quartzite, a metamorphic rock formed from grains of sand cemented in a nonporous fashion—unlike sandstone, which is porous.

LENGTH & CONFIGURATION:
2.7-mile loop

DIFFICULTY: Moderate to difficult

SCENERY: High cliffs, forest, lake

EXPOSURE: Shaded along the top of the bluff, sun along the lake

TRAFFIC: Moderate

TRAIL SURFACE: Mostly asphalt, some rocks, dirt, and roots

HIKING TIME: 1 hour

DRIVING DISTANCE: 34 miles from US 12 and University Avenue

ACCESS: 6 a.m.–11 p.m. year-round

MAPS: USGS *Baraboo;* in the park guide available in the park office; posted at trailhead

WHEELCHAIR ACCESSIBILITY: None

FACILITIES: Restrooms, water, concessions, shelters and picnic area, campgrounds

CONTACT: dnr.wi.gov/topic/parks/name/devilslake, 608-356-8301

COMMENTS: Devil's Lake requires some care and common sense. Several people have fallen to their deaths from the cliffs. Stay on trails and do not climb. Leashed dogs allowed. All vehicles require a park sticker ($7 daily, $25 annual for vehicles with WI plates). Devil's Lake State Park is part of the Ice Age National Scientific Reserve, so vehicle fees are waived for holders of Federal passes. The park participates in the Junior Ranger/Wisconsin Explorer program (see Preface, page 8).

The rock buckled up millions of years ago to form the two ridges. Fast-forward to the most recent glacier of the Ice Age. The ice filled in the valley between the bluffs; when the glaciers retreated, moraines were left at either end, creating the bowl for the lake.

If you put the château between you and the north beach, look for the asphalt path before the château, running left to right. Take it heading west, parallel to the beach and toward the west bluff. It comes to a juncture that goes at an angle left or at an angle right. Take the right branch and follow it to the trees. The trail becomes a wide, crushed-rock path that goes in the direction of the park entrance and parallel to the incoming park road. You come to a map board and a bench on the left. Continue past to another map board at the bottom of a long series of steps up to the left, 0.1 mile from the trailhead. Here's where the climbing begins, quickly giving you some altitude on the park road.

The stairs go 400 feet, and the trail becomes a roughly laid strip of asphalt from here all the way to the descent on the other side of the bluff. Another 100 feet brings you to a bench, and as you keep climbing, you find another bench 0.1 mile later at an observation point. You start to get views of the lake to the east in various places all along the top of the bluff. The path goes over a small rise after this, and you come to some steps 400 feet from the bench. Step up to a rock platform and then down again on the other side. Pass through a rock gateway on stone steps 100 feet later. Another 150 feet brings you to more steps up and over a hump and down the other side, where you continue another 0.2 mile before you find another bench. Another 150 feet past this is a clearing where you can find more benches and a call box. This is for emergencies, and there is a park access road that comes up the west side of the bluff for emergency vehicles.

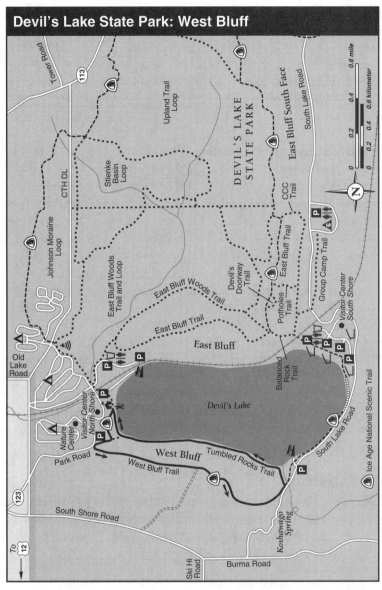

Devil's Lake State Park: West Bluff

Look for a good vantage point to the left here. Continuing along the trail, pass another bench 150 feet later, and then arrive at another good observation point on the left 300 feet beyond that. Another 0.15 mile later is the next good place to perch and look out over the lake, and it is arguably the best overlook on this bluff. A wide, flat expanse of rock makes a natural observation deck from which you can look straight across to the equally open and prominent top-of-the-bluff lookout on the other side. You can see the south shore beach area and the moraine that bridges the southern ends of the two bluffs to close off the lake area.

The trail heads back into the woods from here and takes 0.5 mile to descend about 500 feet in elevation. The last stretch is about 0.1 mile of asphalt with long steps formed into it. At the bottom, find a map board. To your right across the park road is a parking lot if you prefer to hike this from the south. You are standing where the park road passing on your right intersects with Cottage Grove Road right before you. Go right if you want to get a look at Koshawago Spring, which flows into the lake under the park road. To continue the trail, turn left on Cottage Grove Road and go 0.35 mile to Tumbled Rocks Trail. This is an easy walk now all the way back to the north shore beach area with the lake nearby on the right, and the sloping collection of fractured rocks—known as talus—that tumbled down from the quartzite bluffs during the repeated freezings and unfreezings of the last Ice Age.

As you return to the north shore beach area, the asphalt trail angles to the right, bringing you back to where you started. This doesn't have the drama of climbing through talus like the East Bluff does, but the views are just as remarkable, and some hikers might not like the exposed feeling of Balanced Rock Trail on the East Bluff face. The Ice Age Trail shares the portion across the top of the bluff and continues around the lake at either end. The north shore beach area has concessions, boat rentals, restrooms, a nice swimming area, and even Wi-Fi in the château.

Nearby Activities

On the way north to Devil's Lake, head east 2 miles on WI 118 just before crossing the Wisconsin River to find Wollersheim Winery (**wollersheim.com,** 608-847-9463). Open daily 10 a.m.–5 p.m., the winery offers tours 15 minutes past each hour. The cost is $3.50.

GPS COORDINATES AND DIRECTIONS
N43° 25' 39.53" W89° 44' 1.25"

From University Avenue in Middleton, go north on US 12 for 31.5 miles to WI 159. Go right 1.2 miles to County Road DL and turn right again. Follow this road 0.3 mile and stay straight at the state park entrance, following the park road 0.7 mile to the parking lot. For the trailhead, follow the asphalt path west just north of the beach area. You will find a path that heads north toward the park entrance on crushed rock. This is the trailhead.

22 Gibraltar Rock State Natural Area

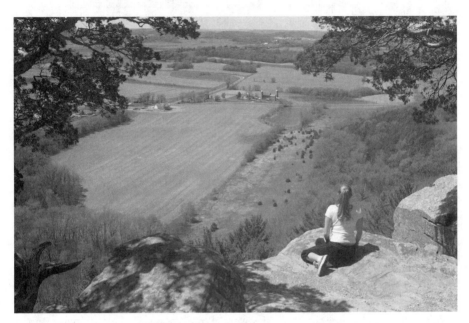

The view from the top of Gibraltar Rock

In Brief

The climb to this extraordinary lookout over the Wisconsin River valley will take your breath away in more ways than one.

Description

This region of Wisconsin is a geologist's dream. From the sandstone of the Cambrian period to the carving work of the glaciers, there is a whole glossary of land features. Gibraltar Rock is a sandstone bluff that rises up out of the earth like a fallen asteroid, and if you aren't ready to exert yourself a bit, this might not be your first hiking choice. Gibraltar Rock is an outlier from the Black River Escarpment. At one time, it must have been attached and then became isolated by erosion. There are others in the area, but this is the highest.

A preservation group called Friends of Our Native Landscape made this park their first project. A famous landscape architect by the name of Jens Jensen led the call to protect this area after the group formed in Madison in 1920. When the land became available in 1927, he and his colleagues, forward thinkers from Madison and the University of

LENGTH & CONFIGURATION:
2.8 miles (1.4 miles, loop only); loop with an optional out-and-back

DIFFICULTY: Moderate to difficult

SCENERY: Mixed forest, cliffs towering over rolling farmland

EXPOSURE: Mostly shaded

TRAFFIC: Light

TRAIL SURFACE: Packed dirt with tree roots, exposed rock, some old asphalt

HIKING TIME: 30 minutes

DRIVING DISTANCE: 1.2 miles from the intersection of WI 113 and County Road V

ACCESS: Year-round

MAPS: USGS *Lodi*

WHEELCHAIR ACCESSIBILITY: None

FACILITIES: None

CONTACT: dnr.wi.gov/topic/lands/naturalareas/index.asp?sna=73, iceagetrail.org, 800-227-0046

COMMENTS: Rock climbing, though popular in the past, is currently prohibited. Pets must be on a leash.

Wisconsin, took action and acquired the deed. The preserved area was first known as Richmond Park, in honor of pioneer couple James and Emma Richmond, who, along with other families, had first homesteaded nearby. You can find a stone marker at the top of the cliff commemorating the preservation group. The 35 acres of Gibraltar Rock were designated a State Natural Area in 1969. A segment of the Ice Age Trail bears the park's name and runs from one parking lot to the other, but this hike as described is a short lollipop using just a portion of the Ice Age Trail segment.

As you enter the parking lot, there is an access road to the left. It's hard to imagine traffic up here, but at one time, vehicles were allowed passage. Efforts to put a stop to underage drinking parties led the park administrators to build the gate you see at the bottom of the hill, and the forest is quickly taking over the access road.

The hike starts at the Ice Age Trail sign at the end of the lot, following a rustic packed-dirt path. Cross the old park road at 350 feet and keep going on a long, slow curve to the top of the bluff. On the left, you'll see a ravine; at 0.2 mile, you cross it on a footbridge. The understory is thin, offering wider views of the terrain.

At 0.6 mile, the trail narrows and takes a turn to go up through some large boulders. To the left you can see the land and trees sloping away. At 0.7 mile, you reach the top of the bluff, but trees still block the view; a cutoff trail to the right takes you back to the former park road. Stay left and gradually the view starts to emerge.

The edge of the cliff is breezy, and those given to vertigo should be warned. Take care here, as there is a lot of loose sand, and the flat stones are less level than you think. Over the years, even a couple of locals who were familiar with the location have fallen to their deaths. Climbing down to lower ledges is not advisable, and, in fact, all rock climbing is prohibited.

To the south is a sheer 200-foot cliff overlooking a large bog and scenic valley. On a clear day, you can see for miles into the Wisconsin River valley and the hazy blue hills of Baraboo. The farmland spreads out before you with the occasional patch of woods here

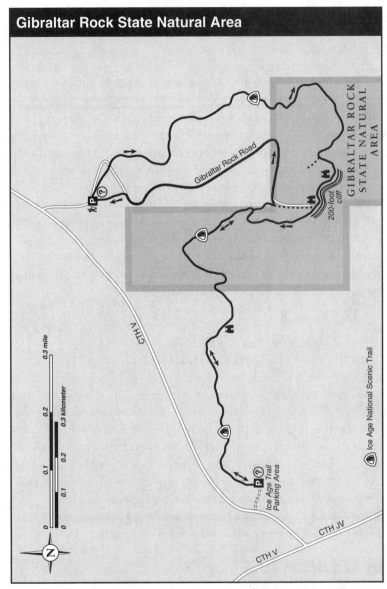

Gibraltar Rock State Natural Area

and there. Migrating raptors are not uncommon; they come here to catch thermals formed by the warm cliff face. Most days you can expect to see turkey vultures riding the up currents and having a look at who's looking at them.

The first lookout area on your right is best for just taking it all in—the sweeping horizon, the circling birds, and the geometric patterns of farmland. Another 200 feet east is another prime lookout point, and this one offers a fine view of the cliff itself, where it juts out from the rest of the bluff and shows off its layered colors of sandstone. This is a good photo angle. The plant life along the cliff is mostly ferns, columbine, and cliff goldenrod. Wildflowers populate the grassy areas set beneath pines, towering red oaks, and cedars.

Most visitors will come for the vista and then just head back down the hill along the former park road turned trail. But the trail beyond, though not as dramatic as the cliffs, offers a moderate challenge and rich plant life. The trail descends over roots and rocks and around a few sizable boulders, a bit challenging at the beginning but becoming less so after the first 300 feet. From here, the trail is still narrow as it passes through thicker undergrowth and tall red oak and basswood. You can expect to have to climb over fallen timber that shows a variety of fungi for the mushroom enthusiasts. You can also find bird's-foot violets and pasqueflowers here in the spring.

Notice a trail juncture on your right, just before you reach a mile of hiking; this is your return path from the out-and-back stretch to the Ice Age Trail parking lot. Go left here and the trail passes under a lot of exposed sandstone.

At 0.3 mile from the juncture, the path heads out into a nice bit of open prairie with views similar to the cliffs but with lower elevation and a feel for the rolling farmland. Just 0.1 mile later, the trail heads back into the woods, continuing to the second parking lot, specifically for the Ice Age Trail, another 0.3 mile later. From here, you must turn around and head back to your return path (unless you drop a second vehicle or bicycle at this lot).

Back at your cutoff point, go left about 200 feet through the woods to that old asphalt road/trail and you have 0.5 mile to get back to the lot. Near the bottom, you will see a rugged trail to the left that cuts directly to the lot, or, if its unstable surface doesn't appeal, continue a short distance to the original bit of trail you came in on.

Gibraltar Rock is a good place to come in late September and early October, when the leaves are turning. The views of the colors below are stunning.

Nearby Activities

Downtown Coffee Grounds is a good place for a cup of joe, some baked goods, and even lunch. It has free wireless Internet access too (107 South Main St., Lodi; 608-592-3325; **facebook.com/downtowncoffeegrounds**).

GPS COORDINATES AND DIRECTIONS
N43° 20' 54.78" W89° 36' 0.75"

From Lodi, go north on WI 113 for 4 miles, then west on CR V for 1 mile, then south (left) on the gravel Park Road 0.2 mile to reach the parking lot.

23 Governor Nelson State Park

Sometimes known as Spring Creek, Dorn Creek flows to Lake Mendota.

In Brief

Explore forest, prairie, savanna, and marshes on the north side of Lake Mendota, and take a swim at the beach afterward with a view of the city across the water.

Description

Former Wisconsin Governor and U.S. Senator Gaylord Nelson is perhaps best known as the founder of Earth Day. A passionate environmentalist, he also helped establish the Apostle Islands as a national lakeshore. This 422-acre state park that bears his name sits across the lake from Madison and is easily accessible.

There are several separate trails throughout the park and, in total, there are 8.4 miles. The selected course starts with the Woodland Trail and takes you through each of the ecological areas. From the northwest corner of the overflow lot, find a map board with nature guides. An access road goes straight past this, but find the trail heading into the woods to your right on a surface of crushed stone.

Boulders are scattered amongst the trees, and flowering bushes and wildflowers are abundant along the path. The understory here is thick and offers no views deeper into the woods.

The trail turns to wood chips less than 100 feet in. You'll find a bench 600 feet from the trailhead and a trail to the right. This is the return for the 1.8-mile Woodland Trail loop. Go straight instead.

LENGTH & CONFIGURATION:
3.9-mile loop

DIFFICULTY: Easy to moderate

SCENERY: Mixed forest, effigy mounds, savanna, prairie, wetlands, stream, lakeshore

EXPOSURE: Mostly sun, parts shaded

TRAFFIC: Light

TRAIL SURFACE: Grass

HIKING TIME: 2 hours

DRIVING DISTANCE: 4.8 miles from University Avenue and Allen Boulevard

ACCESS: 6 a.m.–11 p.m. year-round

MAPS: USGS *Waunakee*; at trailheads and park office

WHEELCHAIR ACCESSIBILITY:
Red-Tailed Hawk Trail; viewing platform; along beach area

FACILITIES: Restrooms, boat landings, fish cleaning station, vending machines, water, pay phones

CONTACT: dnr.wi.gov/topic/parks/name/govnelson, 608-831-3005

COMMENTS: There is a designated dog swim area; otherwise, your pet must be on a leash. Carryout garbage and recycle bags are available at trailheads. A state park vehicle registration sticker (daily or annual) is required. Hiking is not allowed when cross-country skiing is possible. No bikes allowed.

The trail is wide and slightly uneven, tilting to the left in some places. After a couple of bends, take the small loop trail left to see a 358-foot-long American Indian mound shaped like a panther. The 800-foot loop takes you through plenty of wildflowers and yet only about 100 feet from residences just outside the park. Where this trail makes the turn to the right, find a bench with a small overhang. On the left side of the trail beyond a wooden fence is the beginning of the mound, which runs parallel all the way back to the main trail. Ancient effigy mounds were built over long periods of time. Most are conical or linear, but this one is apparently a panther. Mounds may have marked boundaries or events or could have been used to communicate to ancestors. They are still sacred to local tribes and thus protected by law. Stop and read the information board at the end of the trail before continuing left on the main trail.

The trail passes through a row of conical mounds 800 feet from here. The Ho-Chunk Nation occupied this area, which connected major communities via trails linking Mendota, Monona, Dejope, Waubesa, and Kegonsa. You'll find more information and a bench right before the mounds. A wooden fence runs alongside the path and then ends where the trail cuts left from the mounds. Just 300 feet from here is a sandy patch and an area open to the sky.

A spur trail cuts left from here and takes you out of the park to a public road, picnic area, and parking lot. Stay right as the trail curves back around the right and starts heading north to a small clearing and then back into the trees. The trail, sandy in spots, starts to climb the hill, and you find a short bench to your right. Go to the top of the hill, where there are four viewing benches and a memorial rock. The view from here over the trees to the right is quite nice, and a few shade trees make this a perfect place to take a break.

From this clearing there are three trails to the left. The far left trail is part of the Oak Savanna Trail and heads south before turning west to run right along the highway. The far right trail is the last section of the Woodland Trail and intersects with Red-Tailed Hawk Trail before returning to the juncture you passed at the beginning of this hike. The central of the three trailheads is yours, and it climbs a steep hill in the sun. This is also Oak Savanna Trail, heading north as it bypasses the last portion of forest. It's listed as the most difficult trail for its rolling hills. Swallows follow you along a wide, mowed path, and some of the birdhouses may be occupied by bluebirds. You can still see and hear the highway from your trail, but it is not so distracting. The name Oak Savanna may be puzzling because you won't see any oaks out here. Current efforts are making headway to remove nonnative plants and reclaim the area as savanna.

As you come over the next smaller hill, there's a bench. To the left, the road actually disappears behind the hill, and you can see farmland to the north. To the south is the forest you've left. You may see alternative trails that do not follow the map; these are cut by the park for various purposes from time to time and often connect to the trail along the highway.

As you cross the prairie, you come to where Red-Tailed Hawk Trail shares the path, continuing in the direction of the park office, forward and to the left of the trail line. Stay left and watch for the trail's namesake. Right next to the trail juncture, look up prairie plants on an informational sign or take a rest on a bench. You can find compass plant, prairie smoke, bergamot, blue stems, Indian grass, yellow coneflower, prairie shrub, and many other wildflowers nearby. July shows a profusion of purple, and milkweed grows just behind the bench.

Just before the park road, the trail crosses the path along the road. Exit through the gate and cross the road to pick up the trail again. You are now on Morningside Trail, which goes directly left to the office—where you'll find a phone, restrooms, parking, and an ATM—and then around the edge of the prairie past a maintenance building, or directly back to the parking lots and picnic area. There is sometimes a mowed path straight across the field as well. Take a soft left to follow a branch of Morningside Trail (the right one of the two on the left, which are labeled as such).

The trail makes a right-bearing curve across the field a quarter mile through open prairie. Some small trees and shrubs start to appear in the field just past the halfway mark. The next intersection offers a trail going left back along the maintenance area trail. Stay right instead, until you come to an exit from the park that goes to the left. There is a small stop sign here. Cross the road, heading toward a bridge; don't take the private drive to the right. Stay on the right side of the road, cross the bridge over Dorn (Spring) Creek, and watch for waterfowl below. This creek feeds into the larger Six Mile Creek farther to your right and then into the lake 0.6 mile from the bridge. On the other side of Dorn Creek, the trail descends to the right from the shoulder of the road.

Go left at the trail juncture if you want to add another 0.5 mile to your hike. The trail follows the road and loops out through the prairie marsh and returns to this spot. The best viewing of waterfowl will be here at the platform to your right, because the trail cannot get close to the marshes on that loop. You hear more than you can see at that point because brush rises up on both sides of the trail and a line of trees stands between you and the marsh.

The observation deck is wheelchair accessible and looks out over Dorn Creek and over Six Mile Creek farther off to the left. An informational sign can help you identify nearby plants, such as white turtlehead, joe-pye weed, duckweeds, horsetails, cattails, great blue lobelia, and arrow-leaf violets. Backtrack to the park and go left once you cross the private drive entrance and reenter the park.

At a juncture where a trail cuts right back to the trail across the center of the prairie, go straight and enter oak savanna worthy of the name. To the left of the trees, cattails grow out of the marsh. Pass a bench and then come out into the sun again. A trail goes right, but stay the course. Pass a stand of oaks to the left, and then follow the turn as it goes left into scrub brush. Around the bend, look for the skeleton of a dead tree. Cross a metal culvert and plastic posts and, beyond that, a patch of willows to the right.

Follow the trail another 0.2 mile as the brush and forest thicken up around you, blocking views in all directions but granting no shade to the trail. At the end of this segment, the trail passes over another culvert. Eighty feet past this, the trail goes right at a trail post and comes into the shade of some maples.

Here to your left is the pet swim area, where there is a small beach and some picnic tables. A map board stands where the trail cuts to the beach.

Continuing past the swim area another 400 feet brings you out of the woods and to the Indianola Beach Playground/Picnic and Concession Area. The path right goes to a parking area and continues as Morningside Trail. There are actually two trails to the left, but one is just a service road and angles back. Stay on the asphalt path to the left. No pets are allowed beyond this point. This area is Indianola Beach, which hosts a concession stand in the summer. Restrooms, a playground, a pay phone, volleyball nets, and a sandy beach round out the offerings. A sign alongside the trail explains the Ho-Chunk circle of life and seasons.

After a dip in Lake Mendota, continue down the asphalt path to get to all the parking lots. If you parked in the overflow lot, you will need to follow this to the end, where you also will find a boat landing and a fish cleaning station to the left.

Nearby Activities

Just a few miles southwest of Governor Nelson State Park is Mendota Park, situated off County Highway M near the intersection of County Highways Q and M near Middleton. The park has 30 campsites and two shelter facilities.

GPS COORDINATES AND DIRECTIONS

N43° 07' 49.96" W89° 26' 10.90"

From University Avenue on the far west side of Madison, go north on Allen Boulevard 1 mile to Century Avenue. Go right at the traffic light; after almost 1 mile, this becomes County Road M. Stay on CR M 3.8 miles from Allen to arrive at the park entrance on your right. Enter the park and follow the road to the very last parking lot—the overflow lot—on your left. The trailhead is at the right corner of the lot near the entrance.

24 Ice Age Trail: Cross Plains Segment

A dolomite rock outcrop along the Ice Age Trail in Cross Plains

In Brief

Follow a loop of the Ice Age Trail that crosses hilltop prairie and oak savanna to descend into a scenic gorge on the other side.

Description

Loops along the Ice Age Trail are somewhat few, but this one right at the edge of the city of Cross Plains can be fashioned into one with just a short distance of residential street to connect the end points. From the trailhead, the trail follows an old asphalt path up the hill beyond the gate of Hickory Hill Conservancy Park. Despite the name, you are going to see more oaks than hickory, as this park features a bit of oak savanna and a restoration project aiming to create more each year. Wildflowers are abundant throughout the hike, especially in the prairie portions.

LENGTH & CONFIGURATION: 2.8-mile loop	from the juncture of US 14/University Avenue and US 12 in Middleton
DIFFICULTY: Easy with a couple of short moderate climbs	**ACCESS:** Year-round
SCENERY: Mixed forest, prairie, oak savanna, wooded ravines	**MAPS:** USGS *Cross Plains; Ice Age Trail Atlas*
EXPOSURE: Half exposed, half shaded	**WHEELCHAIR ACCESSIBILITY:** None
TRAFFIC: Light	**FACILITIES:** None
TRAIL SURFACE: Packed dirt, grass	**CONTACT: iceagetrail.org,** 800-227-0046
HIKING TIME: 1–1.5 hours	**COMMENTS:** Leashed dogs allowed. Dispersed camping allowed in designated area for thru-hikers only.
DRIVING DISTANCE: 7.9 miles west	

The steepest part of the hike is this asphalt road, and it rises up to a curve to the left 500 feet into the park, where it gradually becomes doubletrack and crushed rock. By a quarter mile, the terrain levels out, and while the doubletrack continues straight, the Ice Age Trail follows a little S-curve to the right (north) into an open prairie full of wildflowers. Just watch for the yellow blazes and arrows that mark the Ice Age Trail. Midway through the field, pass a post where a cutoff trail runs 200 feet to the return trail. Stay straight/left at this juncture and the trail crosses on grass until it reaches the edge of the woods of the S.B. Andersen Memorial Preserve at 0.7 mile. Just inside the trees is a spur trail to the left marked by blue blazes. This is a 250-foot dead-end trail to the Dispersed Camping Area. Camping is for thru-hikers only and limited to one night. There are no facilities. See Dispersed Camping rules on page 13.

Past the camping trail, the trail descends through the forest with thin understory, allowing wider views of the terrain. Stay on the trail as it skirts private land. The path snakes along the edge of a ridge and enters what the trail makers call Three Gorges. This scenic system of ravines and gullies is shaded by old hardwoods, and the path comes down to a footbridge across the bottom of the gorge at 1.1 miles. The trail bears left on the other side but soon switches back as it heads back uphill. At 1.4 miles, you come back out into prairie restoration.

Cross the field, passing a row of trees and brush, and then you are back in the prairie you first crossed. At 1.5 miles, you pass that cutoff trail on your right, an option to turn this into a lollipop trail and head back to the trailhead. But stay left and the trail bends slightly left, heading into oak savanna 200 feet later. The trail angles across the savanna's edge and heads into thick woods at 1.6 miles, where you will find some hickory trees have joined the oaks. Watch for jack-in-the-pulpit and mayapples. A spur trail at 1.8 miles descends to the right into the cul-de-sac on Lewis Street, but continue straight as the trail starts to show a lot more broken rock or glacial till. At 2.2 miles is a bench at the top of the ridge, overlooking Cross Plains. From here, the trail follows switchbacks with stone steps

Ice Age Trail: Cross Plains Segment

A scenic overlook from the Ice Age Trail just above Cross Plains

and some rail-tie and earth steps down through black walnuts. Columbine and other wildflowers are common here.

The trail comes out behind residences and straddles a property line to take you out to Lewis Street, where there are no sidewalks. Go right, and then take a left on Cross Street, which takes you one long block to Hickory Hill Street, where you turn right to find the trailhead again.

Nearby Activities

The Ice Age Trail Alliance keeps its headquarters here in Cross Plains at 2110 Main St. While this isn't a typical visitor center, hikers are encouraged to stop and say hello. Restrooms and water are available, as are showers and laundry facilities for thru-hikers. A lovely rain garden is on site, and more information and Ice Age Trail merchandise are available inside. The offices are open on weekdays 8 a.m.–5 p.m.

GPS COORDINATES AND DIRECTIONS
N43° 7' 6.62' W89° 39' 7.52"

Leaving Madison/Middleton, University Avenue becomes US 14 from its juncture with US 12. Go west 7.6 miles into Cross Plains and turn right (north) on Hickory Street. Drive 0.2 mile and take the second left on Hickory Hill Street. Parking is at the end of the short road, where you will also find the trailhead.

25 Ice Age Trail: Devil's Lake Segment

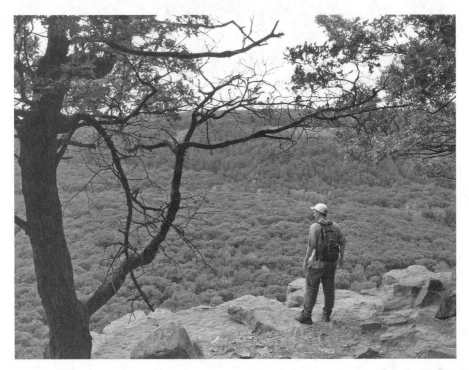

Crossing the east bluff at Devil's Lake

In Brief

Simply the grandest of the area's Ice Age Trail segments, with two dramatic bluffs overlooking Devil's Lake and an assortment of glacial formations, this hike offers a bit of everything and ends at the entrance to Parfrey's Glen, a wonder in its own right.

Description

For me, this is the mother of all the Ice Age Trail segments in the area. The length alone might discourage some hikers or at least compel them to cut it in half, perhaps spending a night camping at Devil's Lake State Park, which is just past the halfway point. If hiked one-way, it requires either two vehicles or a bike drop at Parfrey's Glen to get back to the trailhead. A walk of about 2.9 miles via CR DL and Marsh Road would also work, making this a 21.1-mile loop. Make sure you know when sundown is and that you start early

LENGTH & CONFIGURATION: Up to 18.2 miles; one-way, but 3 miles on road creates a loop of 21.1 miles

DIFFICULTY: Moderate to difficult

SCENERY: Glacial moraines, towering cliffs, hardwood forest, Devil's Lake, creeks, prairie

EXPOSURE: Half and half, but long stretches of shade

TRAFFIC: Light, but potentially moderate to heavy within Devil's Lake State Park bluff areas

TRAIL SURFACE: Packed dirt with roots and rocks, rough asphalt and crushed rock inside the park

HIKING TIME: Up to 8 hours

DRIVING DISTANCE: 36.3 miles from the intersection of US 12 and University Avenue/US 14 on Madison's west side

ACCESS: State park segment's hours are 6 a.m.–11 p.m. year-round

MAPS: USGS *Baraboo*; *Ice Age Trail Atlas*;

Devil's Lake State Park office has maps of the park portions.

WHEELCHAIR ACCESSIBILITY: Only a shoreline portion at Devil's Lake State Park

FACILITIES: Within the state park are restrooms, water, concessions, boat rentals, shelters, and grills. Pit toilets and water at the Parfrey's Glen Natural Area.

CONTACT: iceagetrail.org or **dnr.wi.gov/ topic/parks/name/devilslake,** 800-227-0046. Devil's Lake State Park only: 608-356-8301

COMMENTS: Leashed dogs allowed. Parts of the trail pass through state parks; all vehicles within the park boundaries require a park sticker ($7 daily, $25 annual for vehicles with WI plates). This is also required at the Parfrey's Glen lot at the end of the trail. Devil's Lake State Park is part of the Ice Age National Scientific Reserve, so vehicle fees are waived for holders of Federal passes.

enough to beat it. One more word of warning: Although I don't consider Devil's Lake dangerous, it does require some care and common sense. Over the years, several people have fallen to their deaths from the cliffs. Stay on the trails and do not climb.

From the trailhead, you enter the woods on a narrow, uneven dirt path marked throughout with yellow swatches on posts and trees. You find mixed hardwoods the first 0.4 mile, and then the path heads north, following the edge of a field. You get a nice view of the surrounding hills. On the other side at 0.3 mile, there is a sign indicating 1 mile to Marsh Road. Go through farmland; just before the road, turn right and go 0.1 mile inside the wire fence to a gate.

Cross the road to a metal gate and the trail sign near four large boulders. Follow the country lane straight, with woods to the left and crops to the right. The lane curves left in front of a small stone cabin, but the trail goes right on grass and zigzags across the field to woods on the other side. As you come to the woods 0.25 mile from the road, the trail goes right along the edge a short distance and then left into tall pines. There's a place to clean your boots and another entry point but no parking. Go left here, continuing through the pines 0.15 mile and out onto a boardwalk through wet prairie. It rises over a creek and brings you to a footpath at the edge of some woods, where you continue moderately uphill.

The next 0.8 mile takes you to CR DL. Along the way, you cross a left-to-right trail in the open fields. Go straight, heading toward open water. An arrow points you left as the

Ice Age Trail: Devil's Lake Segment

trail bends around the marshy area. The path heads downhill around a clump of savanna and then over the top of it. Pass over the moraine here as the trail goes right and steeply downhill with the direction of the ridge. A trail sign sends you right, where there is a prairie loop to the left if you want to linger a bit. Head north and cross a small footbridge, climb the next hill to a map board and trail info, and then finish the connection to CR DL.

Cross and go right along the edge of the road until you reach a metal gate with a NO HUNTING sign and a little trail arrow on a post. Squeeze around the end of the gate. The trail goes right on crushed stone and bends left 200 feet down as it crosses a field to another trail arrow. Through a gate on the other side, go left on a grassy trail down a corridor between trees 0.25 mile to WI 113. From there, you can see the bluffs of Devil's Lake. Cross the highway to a parking lot. This is the state park now and would require a vehicle sticker. The trail continues past the lot through Roznos Meadow 1 mile to South Lake Road. You'll find the soil along the way is sandy from the deposits of the glaciers and the prairie has been restored to its early-1800s conditions. You will likely see bluebirds. Beyond to the west, you can see the cliffs and their characteristic talus, sloping rock fragments made by repetitive thaws and freezes during the glacial period. Between the two bluffs is a lower moraine. This moraine, along with the one to the north of the lake, dammed what was once a river and helped form the lake when the glaciers retreated.

At South Lake Road, find another parking lot to the right—another optional starting point, but also requiring a park sticker. From the road, the trail climbs up the side of a ravine at a moderate to difficult grade. The path crosses it at 0.5 mile through a lot of exposed rock under good canopy. At 1.1 miles from the road, come to a bench and a trail juncture. To the right is the Uplands Trail, and you could take it to bypass the entire lake area and bluffs, if you prefer to save those for another day. Go left and continue climbing 0.4 mile from the juncture, where you'll find a bench and scenic overlook and then a spur trail left to rock-climbing areas at 0.15 mile after that. The trail then curves away from the cliff and starts downhill on crushed rock. From the spur trail to the next juncture is 0.5 mile, where you will see the East Bluff Woods Trail and Uplands Trail going to the right. Stay straight for 0.2 mile, and then the trail breaks left from the park trail at a red sign for Moldy Buttress, a rock-climbing point. Follow this path 100 feet out to the cliff on East Bluff Trail. A Civilian Conservation Corps trail goes left here, but go right on an uneven strip of asphalt. You will likely start to see a lot more trail traffic from this point on until you leave the state park.

Continue along the cliff path 0.3 mile to a stone-step trail left down to The Potholes if you want a look at unique erosion patterns formed long ago by swirling rocks in glacial runoff. Just past this trail is a map board, and another 100 feet farther along is another trail down to the left that takes you through the Devil's Doorway. On the other side of this, continue 0.2 mile to the meeting of several trails at a map board at the top of the Balanced Rock Trail. There is an emergency call box here. Look left to a rock ledge overlooking the lake and southern beach area. Look for a trail marker that leads down to the right from here, and follow the 0.3-mile Balanced Rock Trail down the cliff face on rock steps and rough patches of asphalt. At the bottom, cross the railroad tracks, pass through the trees

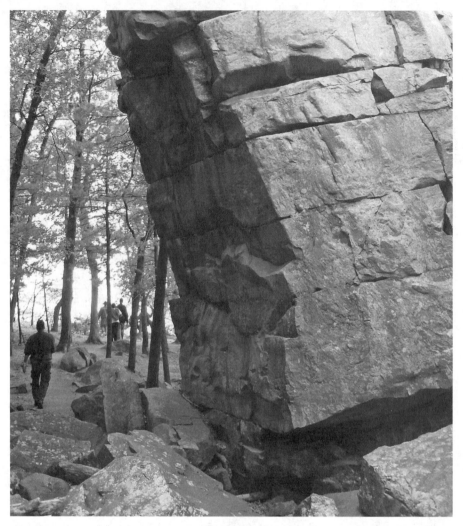

Rock formations along the East Bluff at Devil's Lake

beyond, and come out into the south shore beach area. There is an American Indian bird-shaped effigy mound to the right. You'll find water, restrooms, a beach for swimming, picnic areas, and concessions along the beach.

From the railroad tracks, the Ice Age Trail (IAT) runs 1.2 miles, following the asphalt path along the shoreline around the southern end of the lake on a boardwalk and then just the park road until it arrives at Cottage Grove Road and the trailhead for the West Bluff. You can skip the climb and walk along the lakeshore by taking the Tumbled Rocks path to the right at the end of Cottage Grove Road. Otherwise, start climbing. It's 0.5 mile to the first overlook at the top of the bluff. From there, you have another 0.9 mile along the top of the bluff and then down the northern end to the park road. Go right, following the trail into the park, past the park office, and east over the railroad tracks at the opposite end of the north shore beach. Follow the trail markers, but essentially take the park road to the Ice Age campground, passing under the highway 1 mile from the West Bluff. Come to an intersection; on the other side, take the trail that angles right, also called the Johnson Moraine Trail. Head up the campground road into the woods, find toilets and water on the left, and take a trail into the woods on the right between campsites 419 and 420. Hike another mile, passing a return trail on the right and continuing to CR DL/WI 113. Cross into the woods on the other side, where you'll find a map board.

At 0.1 mile, the Uplands Trail goes straight and right; go left on the IAT, crossing four bridges in 1 mile before arriving at a juncture. The Uplands Trail is to the right; your trail is to the left. Pass another spur trail to a parking lot before you arrive at CR DL/WI 113. Cross at an angle to the left to find the next trail segment. This is 4.2 miles from Parfrey's Glen. The trail is rugged once more, with tree roots and rocks, passing intermittently through mixed forest and prairie and rising and falling with the hills. Two miles from the highway, come to a blue-blazed spur trail to the right (south); this leads a quarter mile out to parking on Solum Lane. But continue east, being careful to follow the yellow arrows and patches. Another 2 miles remain. This path takes you in and out of the woods and prairie uphill for a bit, but then it is mostly downhill through hardwood forest to the end. A few patches show some tricky footing, especially when the light gets low close to sundown, which may be hastened a bit by the hills behind you.

If you have time and energy, do not miss Parfrey's Glen to your left at the end of the trail. The 0.7-mile hike into a unique gorge holds some rare sights in terms of geology, flora, and fauna.

Nearby Activities

On your way here or home, take the free car ferry across the Wisconsin River at Merrimac (considered the only nonwalking segment of the Ice Age Trail). Buy some ice cream at the stand next to the dock on the Merrimac side before the ride over. The ferry shuts down for winter; otherwise, it usually runs 24 hours a day, seven days a week. Watch for flashing signs on US 12, CR K, I-90/94, and WI 60, 19, and 113, which indicate when the ferry is not running.

GPS COORDINATES AND DIRECTIONS
N43° 23' 9.51" W89° 38' 34.13"

From its intersection with University Avenue/US 14, go north 23.2 miles on US 12 to Sauk City. After the bridge over the Wisconsin River, turn right on WI 78 and go 11.8 miles to Merrimac. Go north on Baraboo Road for 0.25 mile. Go left on Cemetery Road for 1 mile (it becomes Marsh Road as you go) and find the trailhead parking lot on your right.

26 Ice Age Trail: Groves-Pertzborn Segment

Passing through a stand of aspen

In Brief

Take a trek through a ravine that lies between two rounded hills set right along the edge of the unglaciated "driftless zone."

Description

The Ice Age Trail is the result of a lot of work by a lot of people. Ray Zillmer, a Milwaukee lawyer, came up with the concept and founded the Ice Age Park and Trail Foundation in 1958. The plan was to make a park not measured in acres but in miles—a serpentine hiking path that would follow the terminal moraine from the last advance of glaciers into

LENGTH & CONFIGURATION: 2.6-mile out-and-back	**DRIVING DISTANCE:** 7.4 miles west from the intersection of I-39 and WI 60
DIFFICULTY: Moderate to difficult	**ACCESS:** Year-round except during gun-hunting season in November
SCENERY: Forest, ravine, some prairie	**MAPS:** USGS *Lodi; Ice Age Trail Atlas*
EXPOSURE: Mostly shaded	**WHEELCHAIR ACCESSIBILITY:** None
TRAFFIC: Light	**FACILITIES:** None
	CONTACT: iceagetrail.org, 800-227-0046
TRAIL SURFACE: Rough dirt path	**COMMENTS:** Beware of poison ivy.
HIKING TIME: 1–1.5 hours	This is a good place to pick berries.

Wisconsin. This is the line where the massive sheets of ice stopped advancing and from which they eventually retreated.

Senator Gaylord Nelson and Congressman Henry Reuss were instrumental in establishing the trail as a national scientific reserve in 1964. In the 1980s, it was designated as both a state and national scenic trail.

Trails are low impact. Nothing is paved, and they are minimally maintained to preserve the natural look of the area. Often you feel as if you are the first person on the trail in a very long time, and it's only the yellow squares posted intermittently on trees and occasional trail posts that reassure you that you are on the right path.

You can thank the myriad volunteers and landowners that helped make this 1,000-mile trail possible. The section you are hiking, in fact, is private property.

Before hiking the trail, check the kiosk for trail news or warnings. There is a map and information on identifying poison ivy. There is enough of it here to warrant posting this warning, so take a moment to make sure you know what it looks like. Wild parsnip can also be found here and is far less infamous than the ivy, but it is arguably much worse.

The trailhead is 30 feet off to the left of the kiosk as you face it. The trail is narrow, and you can expect tree roots and uneven dirt surface. It curves left; 300 feet down the trail, you enter a rather thick stand of aspens. Aspens often clump like this because, unlike seed-producing trees, they actually spread via shoots from the root system. These colonies are considered one single entity, and a particularly large colony of aspens in Colorado is alleged to be the largest living thing on the planet. They are aggressive but native to Wisconsin. Their white or silverfish trunks create a contrast in the darker forest for a nice visual effect.

Throughout this stretch, find black raspberries (known locally as blackcaps) along the trail. They are a bit less sweet than raspberries and usually are ripe as early as late June on into mid-July.

The trail continues uphill on a moderate grade. There's a bench 0.3 mile from the trailhead. At the crest of the hill, only another 300 feet from here, enter a small meadow with wildflowers. To your right are agricultural fields, typically cornfields.

Ice Age Trail: Groves-Pertzborn Segment

Cross this open area and reenter the trees. There's a large boulder on your left; soon after that, the trail begins to descend just a bit. In the spring, this is a good place to find jack-in-the-pulpit and mayapple, and several fern species populate the understory.

The climb resumes 500 feet past the boulder. In another 0.2 mile, cross a private access road that comes up the hill from your left and leads to the crops 100 feet to your right. Continue across another 400 feet and come to a grassy area to the right. The trail continues past, heading through another stand of aspens.

Climb only a bit more, and then come over the ridge and look down into a marvelous ravine. Mayapples are in abundance here. The *Ice Age Trail Guidebook* compares this to a rain forest, and truly there is something of the ravine that does give the feeling you are not in Wisconsin. Woods with thick brush often close in around you and give the impression you could be anywhere. When a space opens up like this under the canopy of oaks and basswoods without a lot of intervening brush, and the landscape folds with a crease between two ridges, it certainly does leave an impression. Watch for owls, and, if you are really lucky, you might see a Cooper's hawk that has been spotted around here.

Follow the trail as it switches back and forth, taking you down into the bottom of the ravine on a moderate grade, and then follow an easterly trail up the opposite side. The slope is not so steep that it should be a concern for falling.

Cross the next ridge and begin your descent to the end of the trail. When you come upon some old power lines, you are actually halfway down the hill. The path shows sandy spots as you pass some cedar. The canopy is thinned out, and you have only partial shade. This is another nice area for picking blackcaps. Beware: They do stain your hands a bit.

The ground is soft and spongy beneath your feet because burrowing creatures, such as moles, are common. As the trail dips into a gully, head left and come up on the other side to Bilkey Road opposite a tree farm.

You could drop off another vehicle here to do this one-way, but the distance is short and the times I've been here, I've seen enough wildlife to make a second pass worth it.

Nearby Activities

Cross the Wisconsin River on the only free ferry in Wisconsin. The Merrimac Ferry operates 24 hours a day taking cars, bicycles, and pedestrians from the eastern bank at Okee to the western side at Merrimac. On the other side, check out the geological wonder that is Parfrey's Glen at the head of the Ice Age Trail segment that connects the site to Devil's Lake State Park.

GPS COORDINATES AND DIRECTIONS

N43° 29' 44.83" W89° 34' 47.41"

From the intersection of WI 60 and WI 113 in the town of Lodi, go north 1.2 miles to County Road J. Head left 1.9 miles to find the parking area for the Ice Age Trail on your left, just before the intersection of CR J and Lovering Road. The trailhead is at the parking lot to the left of the trail kiosk.

27 Ice Age Trail: Lodi Marsh Segment

The prairie loop

In Brief

Follow a guided nature loop across a hilltop prairie overlooking the marsh, and then climb a bluff through forest and restored prairie with views of rolling farmland.

Description

Lodi Marsh and its springs surround the upper 2 miles of Spring Creek. They are breeding grounds for several species of birds, including great blue herons, sandhill cranes, willow and alder flycatchers, and blue-winged warblers. If you are into moths—and who isn't?—this is a moth-rich environment, several of which are found only in wetlands.

LENGTH & CONFIGURATION: 7.8-mile loop and out-and-back	**ACCESS:** Year-round
DIFFICULTY: Moderate	**MAPS:** USGS *Lodi; Ice Age Trail Atlas*
SCENERY: Prairie, mixed forest, and bluffs	**WHEELCHAIR ACCESSIBILITY:** None
	FACILITIES: None
EXPOSURE: Half and half	**CONTACT: iceagetrail.org,** 800-227-0046
TRAFFIC: Light	**COMMENTS:** Leashed dogs allowed May 1–July 31. The northernmost portion of the trail is closed during the 9-day deer-hunting season at the end of November. There is an alternative trail exit at Riddle Road. The marsh loop has a corresponding nature trail guide in a box at the trailhead.
TRAIL SURFACE: Cut-grass paths, narrow packed-dirt trails	
HIKING TIME: 3 hours	
DRIVING DISTANCE: 24 miles from I-39 and US 151	

Some rare species include the silphium borer moth, Newman's brocade, and the ottoe skipper. On the south side of the marsh is a 240-foot knob hill partly covered with dry-mesic forest composed primarily of red oak, sugar maple, and basswood. The south slope, however, is prairie.

This segment of the Ice Age Trail has two parts. The first is a 1.5-mile lollipop out through the knob-hill prairie that borders the wetlands west of the trailhead parking lot. The second stretch is one-way or out-and-back heading east from the marsh trailhead and lot to WI 113 just south of Lodi. At the little turnaround-cum–parking lot, there is a trail kiosk and a map box that occasionally has maps and the nature trail companion in it. From the lot, head west descending into prairie. You'll find an abundance of wild berga-mot, but beware of the wild parsnip that leans into the trail at times. If the trail has recently been mowed and you're not wearing closed footwear, there is a higher risk of getting exposed to the parsnip juices.

At 0.15 mile, you enter oak savanna. The trail then passes along a ridge, with a steep slope down to the right where you can see flowing water. The trail curves left 0.2 mile later and enters a clearing. Far to the left is rolling farmland. Continue another 0.2 mile to the fork for the loop. Go right up the hill and through partial shade for 0.3 mile, where the trail descends to the turnaround another 0.1 mile later. The trail comes back 0.4 mile to an access road that runs left to right. Stay right. Look for the trail post with the yellow swatch on it to avoid taking intermittent maintenance or prairie restoration paths. The trail climbs over the hump to the north to reconnect with the inbound stem. Go right and return to the parking lot.

From the parking circle, cross Lodi-Springfield Road and find the next segment of the trail to the right. This is the trailhead for the East Lodi Marsh Segment. It starts uphill through prairie and then heads into mixed forest after 0.25 mile. The canopy is thick here, and the packed dirt path curves around the crown of the bluff until a trail marker leads right at 0.1 mile with a view out to a valley and farmland. The path reenters the trees,

Ice Age Trail: Lodi Marsh Segment

mostly aspens, and switches back downhill along a gorge before arriving at a bridge 0.35 mile away. A second bridge is just several steps past that.

From here, the trail opens to the sky for the next 1.1 mile before you hit woods again. Initially, you are surrounded by brush, and you climb a grassy path uphill, offering more views of farmland in the distance. The path winds through open prairie then, offering an easy climb higher and higher on the hill. Follow the posts across the field when the path is not clear, as may be the case after a restorative prairie burn. On the opposite end is a farmhouse and barn; the trail heads toward them. Pass behind a row of trees to enter another field. The trail goes right at a trail sign with brush on either side, and then it heads downhill to a bench on the left with a trail sign and mileage to Lodi: 2 miles. You're actually only 1 mile from the parking lot at the end of this segment, however.

Most of this stretch is downhill through oak-hickory forest with some exposed rock in the surrounding terrain. The trail is a narrow, packed-dirt footpath with tree roots and scattered rocks, becoming rockier and steeper as you go. At 0.5 mile, you come to a spur trail to the left. This takes you 0.15 mile out to Riddle Road. This exit trail must be used during deer season at the end of November, when the last portion of this trail is closed.

Just past the exit trail is an ATV trail crossing left to right, and this is where you see the hunting warning. Past here, follow a 0.15-mile narrow corridor of trees and brush surrounded by agricultural fields. At the end, the trail heads to the right into the sun and borders the fields as it heads east. Watch for trail posts. As you pass through a break in the trees, there will be one ahead and to the right. This will lead you to a crushed-rock road to the left; don't go right. You'll pass under a viaduct at 0.2 mile and then continue up the road to the parking lot 0.1 mile from there. Pass through a gate and go left to the lot. Lodi is 0.4 mile north of here on WI 113. The Ice Age Trail does continue into town on sidewalks and paths. It will eventually connect to the Groves-Pertzborn Segment on the other side of town.

Nearby Activities

On Main Street in downtown Lodi, you can find Suzy the Duck. Spring Creek passes under the street here and waterfowl frequent the area. You can feed them with food from a nearby vending machine. Suzy is the nickname for whichever duck happens to build its nest in a small stone basket here. Look for cafés, coffee shops, and a bakery along Main Street.

GPS COORDINATES AND DIRECTIONS
N43° 16' 55.22" W89° 32' 49.37"

From where it intersects with US 151, take I-39 north from Madison 16 miles to Exit 119 (Lodi/Arlington). The exit loops, and you go right (west) 4.4 miles on WI 60 to reach Lodi. From the intersection of WI 60 and 113 (Main Street and Portage Street) in Lodi, take WI 60 west 0.6 mile. Turn left on Riddle Road, also known as Lodi-Springfield Road. There is a kiosk 3 miles from here on the right side of the road and an area for parking right at the trailhead.

28 Ice Age Trail: Table Bluff Segment

A scenic overlook along the trail

In Brief

Enjoy some rather stunning prairie reclamation where wildflowers abound, and then hike over hills and farmland to a scenic overlook.

Description

This segment of the Ice Age Trail opened in the fall of 2006, and the prairie segments are awash with color when the wildflowers are in bloom. The trail is marked with posts with arrows or trees with plastic yellow patches and is maintained by volunteers. The parking lot is a grassy area along the south side of the road surrounded by several large rocks. The trailhead is clearly marked.

Start along a mowed path through prairie, which soon gives way to a bit of oak savanna. Far to your right is a red barn and farmhouse. The trail heads down the hill into a small hollow and climbs back up at a moderate grade. Watch for a trail to the right marked by white blazes, not yellow. This alternative path runs 0.5 mile along a wooded ridge with views of the valley to the east. Consider it for the return trip because this next

LENGTH & CONFIGURATION: 5-mile out-and-back	**ACCESS:** Year-round, but the privately owned section is closed during the nine-day gun-hunting season in November.
DIFFICULTY: Moderate to difficult	
SCENERY: Prairie, bluffs, mixed forest, farmland, and a scenic overlook	**MAPS:** USGS *Black Earth*
EXPOSURE: Half and half	**WHEELCHAIR ACCESSIBILITY:** None
TRAFFIC: Light	**FACILITIES:** Pavilion, portable toilet
TRAIL SURFACE: Mowed grass, packed dirt, rugged	**CONTACT: iceagetrail.org,** 800-227-0046
	COMMENTS: Leashed dogs allowed. Much of this terrain is private land, and the limited facilities are privately owned as well, though available for use.
HIKING TIME: 2 hours	
DRIVING DISTANCE: 8.3 miles west of the intersection of US 14 and US 12	

stretch of prairie is the best of the bunch, overflowing—especially in the summer—with a wide range of native wildflowers: wild bergamot, black-eyed Susans, gray-headed and purple coneflowers, false sunflowers, Culver's root, butterfly weed, stiff gentian, hoary vervain, prairie smoke, pasqueflowers, and leadplant, just to name a few.

On the other side of this 0.2-mile section, the trail heads into a forest predominantly populated with hickory and oak along a rough dirt path. You are skirting a ridge that slopes to the left into thick underbrush. Watch for rocks and tree roots on the trail.

After a switchback, the trail surface is not always level and sometimes slopes right with the hill itself. You come to a curve with a fence to your left. The trail goes right out of the woods under a large maple. To the left is private property, so do not take the trail there that may be the most obvious path, depending on recent maintenance or traffic. Stay right; if the grass is overgrown, look straight ahead for the post with the yellow patch on it that marks the trail. Cross here along the edge of a farmer's field until you reach scattered trees. A trail marker indicates left. At the other side of this small clearing, head back into the woods. The white-blazed trail connects here from the right as well.

A sign here explains the conditions laid out so that we the public could have access to this segment of the trail. Private owners have granted an easement that does not allow motorized vehicles. You may, however, come across people associated with the property owners who are allowed to use vehicles here. The segment from this point to the southern end of the trail is closed during deer hunting season in November.

The trail climbs over packed dirt with a slope to the left, and in some places rocks have been laid at the edge to maintain the trail and prevent erosion. At the crest of the hill, there is a bench on the left. This area is more open like savanna but then becomes thick woods again for the descent. The trail crosses a gully at the bottom and then bears left along a barbed-wire fence. There is a small rise and another descent that brings you to a small wooden bridge with railings over another gully with a bit of water running through it. From here, the trail heads up again.

Ice Age Trail: Table Bluff Segment

A compass plant in the prairie restoration

Listen for the outbursts of crows, or maybe the screech of a hawk over the nearby prairies, if you're lucky. There are patches of fern here, and because the understory is thick, you may hear more deer than you see. Just past the summit of this next bluff, a private access road crosses the path. Keep straight and watch for the trail post there. Stands of aspen start to appear in the surrounding woods, as well as much smaller oaks and hickory than before.

Don't be startled if you see a small bikini-clad gator lounging to the left side of the path. Just beyond this, the trail joins an access road and goes right on a wide, two-tire path through the woods. Come around the bend into a small clearing, and head straight across.

It is breezier up here along the top of the bluff, and you enter another patch of prairie full of wildflowers. Pass along its right side and enter into partial shade where, in July, you'll find lots of raspberries and blackcaps.

You will find another white-blazed parallel trail on your left, which you can either hike now or as an alternative return path. Oak and hickory savanna holds the top of the hill, and as you pass through the grassy area beneath the trees, you get a bit of sunlight. Emerging around you is the view of the rolling topography of the Driftless Area below and in the distance. Farms poke up from forested areas tucked among hills and swatches of cornfields.

The white-blazed trail joins again from the left just before you reach a clearing. There's often a portable toilet here to the right in this clearing as you come out of the trees, and to the left is a pavilion with picnic tables, which the property owners have kindly allowed hikers to use, so long as they do so responsibly. The owners reserve the right to unobstructed use. There are receptacles for trash and recyclables. The view of the surrounding land from the top of this hill is wonderful.

Continue walking, heading into tall grass and scattered oaks. To your left and below are some marshland and a couple of ponds. The path is steep through oaks, with rocky outcroppings to the left often blocking the view. When you come to a private land sign to the right, bear left and the trail will appear to come to the edge of a cliff. Until you are right upon it, you don't see the path that switches back on dirt and scattered stones, keeping the outcroppings to the left and wildflowers to the right. This is the most charming spot on the trail. Stone steps help you make the next switchback. The trail descends back across the ridge to an arrow that sends you straight down the hill past some smaller oaks. Take the short boardwalk across a marshy spot to access the road from the southern end of the trail segment. A cable across the road prevents car access. The road up to the left is private.

This access road, with prairie grass to the right and cattails to the left, leads to Scheele Road. Left from there leads to CR KP. You can park here, as well as along the east side of the road—maybe you'll have a second car to do the trail one-way—but hikers are encouraged to use the designated lot at the trailhead on Table Bluff Road. A map here shows you the way to the northern end.

Eventually, this trail connects to the nearby Cross Plains segment of the Ice Age Trail.

Nearby Activities

Arguably the best shoe store in the Madison area and a good source for hiking boots is The Shoe Box in nearby Black Earth on US 14 and Mills Street. Stop by or call 608-767-3447.

GPS COORDINATES AND DIRECTIONS

N43° 08' 38.59" W89° 40' 13.29"

Go west on US 14 for 8.3 miles from where it crosses US 12. Just past Cross Plains, take County Road KP north 2.4 miles to Table Bluff Road. Go left 0.3 mile to the small grass parking area and trailhead on the left side of the road.

29 Indian Lake County Park

The trail skirts along the shore of Indian Lake.

In Brief

Sign in as a visitor in a historic chapel on a bluff overlooking a small lake, and then hike parts of the Ice Age Trail and local ski trails over rolling hills.

Description

In the winter of 1856, John Endres and his entire family became infected with diphtheria during an epidemic in southern Wisconsin. The disease was especially dangerous for children, and Endres climbed to the top of the hill above their home and prayed, promising that if his family survived, he would construct a chapel there. Indeed, everyone survived, and Endres made good on his promise. In 1857, he constructed the tiny St. Mary of the Oaks, containing an altar with a praying Virgin Mary, a picture of Jesus, and various other religious objects. Hikers can—and often do—sign the guest book there.

It is arguably the main attraction at this 453-acre county park, where a portion of the Ice Age Trail skirts a small lake left by retreating glaciers. In fact, a segment of the Ice Age Trail is also located in this park, and the path I mapped out contains a portion of that, in addition to some of the great trails deeper in the woods.

LENGTH & CONFIGURATION: 4.7-mile loop	**MAPS:** USGS *Black Earth* and *Springfield Corners;* map board at trailhead
DIFFICULTY: Easy to moderate	**WHEELCHAIR ACCESSIBILITY:** Grassy paths around the lake
SCENERY: Hilly woods, a historic chapel, prairie, and a small lake	**FACILITIES:** Restrooms, pavilion, picnic tables
EXPOSURE: Half shaded, half exposed	**CONTACT:** countyofdane.com/lwrd/ parks/indian_lake.aspx
TRAFFIC: Light	
TRAIL SURFACE: Grass, packed dirt	**COMMENTS:** Dogs can be unleashed in the designated area, but owners must pay a fee at the self-pay station in the parking lot to the west just off the highway. Portions of this park are part of the Ice Age Trail, and the cross-country skiing trails are excellent and challenging.
HIKING TIME: 2–2.5 hours	
DRIVING DISTANCE: 2.2 miles west on WI 19 from US 12	
ACCESS: 7 a.m.–10 p.m.	

In the parking lot, there are pit toilets, and nearby is a pavilion with a few picnic tables. At the south end of the parking lot, find a map board, which marks the head of the Ice Age Trail segment. But don't start here; rather, follow the edge of the parking lot left from here and walk to the edge of the woods to the trailhead. A boardwalk and steps start up the hill for the first 100 feet toward the chapel, and then the trail becomes crushed rock.

Cross an access road that runs left to right and continue up the hill. Expect a bit of huffing and puffing. Another 500 feet up, the slope through oak and hickory forest brings you to an intersection where a trail goes to the right over an unshaded swell. Stay left for now, though you will be returning for this other branch after your visit to the top of the hill. Just past here are a few more steps and then a boardwalk. Toward the top of the hill, the trail becomes packed dirt through an area rather good for raspberries in July. The trail does a turn back to the left and brings you to the chapel. Many visitors find a bit of peace up here in the woods, although the Catholic affiliations draw protests from those who don't feel a religious site should be maintained within a public county park.

The trail continues past the chapel and out onto a cliff, where there's a nice lookout over the lake below. Sit on the bench here amid wildflowers, and take in the view of lake and rolling farmland and forest.

Go back down the hill to the intersection at the end of the boardwalk, and go left along the top of a ridge with slopes to either side. Go left off the top of the ridge just before a large oak, where the path takes you down a steep and narrow footpath and to open prairie. If you went right at the large oak up top, you would descend to the access road you crossed earlier. But the path you are on also rejoins the access road and a mowed area 500 feet from the top of that ridge. Straight ahead are a couple of picnic tables and a log cabin shelter used as a warming house in winter. Part of the Ice Age Trail is straight ahead and slightly to the left, going to the left of some trees that separate it from the shelter area. To the right is part of that access road. Instead, go left at this juncture and follow

Indian Lake County Park

The scenic overlook near the famous Saint Mary of the Oaks chapel

the long trail around the back of the park, with plenty of woods and a hilly terrain, before coming out on the other side in prairie and overlooking the lake.

Your trail has a wooden post marker that reads #1. Cross the field until you reach the trees at 600 feet. This is a nice stretch for prairie flowers in the spring and summer, especially bird's-foot violets in spring. The trail passes into a clump of trees for 300 feet before returning to the open prairie. Another 800 feet later, a line of trees begins to the right. Beyond this, as the trail begins to curve right with the edge of the forest, find a bench on your left. The trail curves all the way back the other direction and enters a forest with a very high and thick canopy. Cross a culvert there; from here, the hiking is typically moderate or a bit more. The trail starts to slope up and follows around a bend through a sharp dip in the terrain and then more climbing. The understory is thin through here, and you really get a sense of the undulating lay of the land beneath the towering trees.

Follow the trail's curve to the right and pass a wooden trail marker not long before you look down to your left into a deep gulley in the woods. From here, the path goes uphill once more. Trees creak in the wind like old rockers or perhaps a ship. At the top of the hill, the terrain slopes down to your right. The trail also descends to a cutoff trail with a marker labeled 2/3, indicating two of the three numbered skiing/hiking trails in the park.

Go left and you will soon encounter a wrong-way sign. Don't worry; this is for cross-country skiers to avoid head-on collisions. Just 200 feet past here is another 2/3 trail marker with a path heading back to the right. Take the soft left following the #2 trail. Again ignore the wrong-way indicator (except during ski season) and pretend you are a rebel. Pass another gulley, this one to the right.

The trail heads to the right, and along here to your left is farmland just 100 feet through the trees. Watch for a posted poem 700 feet along a rather straight stretch until you come to a bend to the left where the trail starts a slow climb and comes to another fork. Stay left again. The trail climbs to your highest point on this hike 0.3 mile later. From here is the steepest descent. Imagine that this is *up*hill for cross-country skiers going the "correct" way. The trail descends about 200 feet in altitude over 0.3 mile. Halfway down, you pass a bench.

From the forest, head into the open, with aspens to your left. Seven hundred feet later, the trail comes to a scenic overlook and bench where there's an intersection with the Ice Age Trail heading left. Read the amusing sign about crows to the right, and take in the view of the lake and prairie. Descend an open field toward the lake, stopping for a break, if you need one, at another bench halfway down.

At the bottom of the hill, the trail goes right back to the parking lot, but continue left to go around the lake. This area of the park has gone to the dogs—literally. Pet owners delight in one of the few areas where they are allowed to unleash the hounds. Benches look out over the lake to the right at a couple of spots along here. Some willows line the water. Trails are cut each year through the field to the left. Stay on the main trail along the lake until it breaks left and crosses the field 700 feet to a bridge where the Ice Age Trail rejoins and crosses Halfway Prairie Creek. Cross and go right until you reach a parking lot on your left. This segment of the Ice Age Trail ends here. This lot is most convenient for hikers with pets. Here you can check another map board and self-pay the dog fee. To your right is a boat landing. Go straight across between the lot and dock, and pick up the trail on the other side. A short way down the trail, pass through a gate. This area offers partial shade under the taller trees that run between the highway to your left and the lake on your right.

You arrive at a farmer's field, most often planted with corn or alfalfa, on your left. On your right, watch for a small point that leans out into the lake. This is a nice spot to watch for waterfowl. Past this point, the grassy trail moves away from the water's edge and becomes marshy. Cattails and willows dominate the surrounding terrain, eventually giving way to cottonwoods before the trail opens up again to the open sky.

This is the lowest segment of the trail; on some older maps, it may even look like you are hiking in the lake. In wet seasons, this path will get soggy. At the corner of the farmer's field, go left, with willows at your right. The trail follows a gentle S around the field's edge and then leads you to the pavement of the park entry road. Follow this back to the parking lot to complete the loop.

Nearby Activities

The Tree Farm is located just a couple of miles west of Indian Lake at 8454 Highway 19 in Cross Plains. They sell Christmas trees for the holiday season but are also an excellent pick-your-own vegetable, herb, and flower farm throughout the growing season. Call 608-798-2286 or go online to find out what's ripe for the picking: **thetreefarm.net.**

GPS COORDINATES AND DIRECTIONS
N43° 11' 22.18" W89° 37' 13.57"

Take US 12 north from Madison to WI 19. Go west 2.2 miles to the park entrance on the left. Follow the park road 0.4 mile to the parking lot. The Ice Age Trail enters on the park road and continues straight at the end of the lot near a map board. The hike outlined here, however, starts to the east of the lot at the bottom of steps that disappear into the woods.

30 Mirror Lake State Park

A view of the lake from Northwest Loop Trail

In Brief

Take the easy way or the more difficult path through the woods along the edge of Mirror Lake. Hike to a scenic overlook when you are done.

Description

From the park office, go west on a gravel trail just north of the visitor center door. The trail crosses the asphalt turnaround near the park entrance. The trailhead is straight across into the woods near a trail marker. The trail on the first loop is easy through pine and mixed forest on a path of mowed grass with some sandy patches.

Just 250 feet into the woods is the first trail juncture and a trail map. Go right to begin the East Loop, or continue straight to get to the less traveled loops to the west. Going right, the trail heads gently downhill through oaks with partial canopy cover and then into evergreens as it slopes up again. At 0.2 mile is the next trail juncture and another map board where a spur trail goes right into the parking lot near the visitor center. From the second map board, it is another 0.5 mile to the turnaround point of this loop. The trail

LENGTH & CONFIGURATION:	WHEELCHAIR ACCESSIBILITY:
3.3 miles (plus a separate 1-mile scenic overlook trail); two loops	A separate trail with a scenic overlook
DIFFICULTY: Easy to moderate	**FACILITIES:** Restrooms, water, campgrounds, playgrounds, swimming beach
SCENERY: Woods, lake overlooks, some exposed sandstone	**CONTACT: dnr.wi.gov/topic/parks/ name/mirrorlake,** 608-254-2333
EXPOSURE: Mostly shaded	**COMMENTS:** All vehicles require a park sticker ($7 daily, $25 annual for vehicles with WI plates). At the visitor center, you can get a checklist for wildflowers, butterflies, and summer birds you may see in the park, plus an educational guide for the Time Warp Trail. The park participates in the Junior Ranger/Wisconsin Explorer program (see Preface, page 8). There are nearly 10 more miles of hiking, biking, and skiing trails inside the park not included in this particular hike/map.
TRAFFIC: Light to moderate	
TRAIL SURFACE: Packed dirt, mowed grass, cedar chips	
HIKING TIME: 1.5 hours	
DRIVING DISTANCE: 45 miles north of the I-39 and US 151 juncture	
ACCESS: 6 a.m.–11 p.m. year-round	
MAPS: USGS *Wisconsin Dells South;* at park office and trail junctures	

turns toward Bluewater Campground and heads back in the opposite direction with no canopy coverage. A spur trail goes right to a picnic area. As you come up on 0.5 mile, you start to see playground equipment as you go up a short hill to the clearing. To your left you see pit toilets and a map board. There is a beach here for swimming. You can get to the Echo Rock Trail from here as well (see below). The return segment of the East Loop is also to your left, just 20 feet away right before the toilets, and it heads back into the woods in the direction you just came. On your right, you pass a playground and a trail to the swimming area. There is no lifeguard. The return segment of the loop is 0.3 mile, and you can see the lake through the trees to your right.

You return to the main trail and a map board. Another 200 feet to your left is the beginning of the East Loop, and it is 0.1 mile back out to the trailhead from here. Go right (west) as the trail comes out of the woods with a nice view of one long finger of Mirror Lake to your right. Cross a small footbridge over a creek into the lake and stay right. A spur trail breaks left out to Fern Dell Road just before the bridge. Just after the bridge to your left is the Time Warp Trail, a 0.4-mile loop you can explore with a corresponding interpretive booklet from the visitor center. Go straight as the next trail juncture begins the next loop, which is a combination of the North, West, and Northwest loops. Go right at the next juncture into the woods under the thick canopy of oaks.

To your right is the lake but with better views in fall and spring when the leaves are gone. At 0.4 mile, the trail bends left as you come to a map board. The trail left is a segment shared by the North and West loops and heads away from the lake into the center of the woods, where you would have a choice to go north on the 1.2-mile North Loop or southwest on the West Loop for a 1.3-mile loop.

Mirror Lake State Park

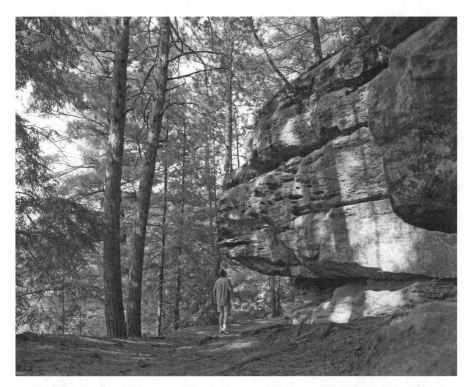

Echo Rock Trail

Staying on this perimeter trail, you find the trail shows some sandy spots and the tree cover becomes smaller maples. The trail bends right and goes uphill moderately until it arrives at a short path to a ledge on the right for a good view of the greater lake at 0.1 mile. The trail descends a bit to another good view 0.1 mile later. The path rises and falls with the terrain, and you cross a crease in the earth that slopes right to the water. The meager understory with lots of dead wood allows you to see the roll of the land and gives you a better chance of spotting deer.

Another 0.1 mile takes you into a clearing where the trail bends right and you see the foundation of an old house to your left. Just past it to the right is a railing along the curving trail with the best views of the water below. The trail rounds the point through a grassy clearing and passes a bench on the left before heading back into pine forest. From here, the grade is moderately uphill on a trail of grass and pine needles. You'll notice two concrete tire paths up the hill, a previous driveway for the cottage you just saw. These continue uphill another 300 feet.

You reach another juncture 0.1 mile from the start of the concrete paths. Go right here, following the arrows. Another 0.1 mile brings you to another juncture and a trail map. The left trail is part of the North Loop. You continue right on the Northwest Loop. This portion of the trail weaves back and forth through the forest and rises up and down like a roller coaster. This is the most difficult section with short, moderate-to-steep climbs. In another 0.2 mile, you see a ridge with exposed sandstone 50 feet to your left. Ferns grow up to the bottom of it. The path climbs steeply, curves left, and then goes directly up to the top of the ridge, where you can see the exposed stone to either side of you.

From the top of the ridge, you have 0.8 mile more of a path going up and down through gullies with good shade. Follow the arrows to stay on the path, because there might be park access roads or old trails visible in the brush. The trail is mostly packed dirt and grass with tree roots, though you may find cedar chips on the steep portions to cut down on erosion. At 0.8 mile, the trail emerges into a clearing. Go straight across to the trees; at 0.1 mile, come to another map board. A trail goes left here right through the middle of the loops. Another trail 300 feet after this goes right out to Fern Dell Road and is the return path of the Time Warp Trail. From the map board if you stay straight, it will take you 0.3 mile out to the trailhead, retracing your steps starting just before you reach the footbridge.

Be sure to go check out Echo Rock Hiking Trail, a 1-mile loop with an optional 0.4-mile out-and-back asphalt segment that is wheelchair-accessible. It is the best scenic overlook of the lake, and the trail from the viewing area down into the woods takes you close to the eroded sandstone. You can drive to the north end of the park and pass the Cliffwood Campground for parking at the trailhead. Another option is to hike there from the northern turnaround point on the East Loop Trail. If you continue straight through the playground/picnic area there and north through the parking lot, a trail will connect you to the concessions area. Follow along the north side of the concessions parking lot to the right, and a paved trail will take you to the trailhead of the Echo Rock Trail. Other park loops include a 0.7-mile interpretive trail to the east and more than 9 miles of bike trails to the south of Fern Dell Road that are also hikeable.

Nearby Activities

The Aldo Leopold Legacy Center (608-355-0279) features exhibits and guided tours for those interested in the life and work of the conservationist and author of *A Sand County Almanac.* It's open Thursdays and Fridays 10 a.m.–4 p.m. and Saturdays noon–4 p.m.

You can see all 15 species of cranes at The International Crane Foundation (E11376 Shady Lane Road, Baraboo; 608-356-9462; **savingcranes.org**).

GPS COORDINATES AND DIRECTIONS
N43° 33' 42.88" W89° 48' 29.71"

From its intersection with US 151, take I-90/94 West 42.5 miles north to US 12/Wisconsin Dells Parkway (Exit 92). Go left (south) 0.6 mile to Fern Dell Road. Turn right (west) and follow this road 1.5 miles to the park entrance. The trailhead is immediately on your left as you enter. Park to your right beyond the visitor center.

31 Natural Bridge State Park

Natural Bridge

In Brief

A magnificent sandstone arch, the largest in the state, is the star of the show, typically overshadowing a nice challenging hike across a neighboring bluff. Educational signage makes this a minicourse in medicinal plants.

Description

This quiet, out-of-the-way state park draws visitors to see its 35-foot-high sandstone arch, but most people don't realize that between 9000 and 8000 B.C., this place was already occupied, making it one of the oldest confirmed settlements in northeastern North America. Archaeologists found artifacts and animal remains—15 different types of mollusks and 50 vertebrates, ranging from passenger pigeon to mountain lion—in and around a rock shelter at the base of the arch. Tribes such as the Fox and the Sauk also occupied the area prior to the arrival of white settlers, but even they are relatively late arrivals.

From the end of the parking lot, look north across the open mowed area, where you see pit toilets to the right and a water pump to the left. There are two trailheads: one directly north near the pump, which offers a short, quick route to the arch, and the trailhead for the hike described here, which is located behind the toilets on the right, not as easy to see.

LENGTH & CONFIGURATION:
2.4-mile loop

DIFFICULTY: Moderate to difficult

SCENERY: Sandstone bluffs, a stone arch, mixed forest, some prairie

EXPOSURE: Mostly shaded

TRAFFIC: Light to moderate near the arch; more deer than people in the southern section

TRAIL SURFACE: Packed dirt, some mowed grass and steps

HIKING TIME: 1–1.5 hours; 30 minutes for just the arch

DRIVING DISTANCE: 10.9 miles west of US 12 on County Road C

ACCESS: 6 a.m.–11 p.m. year-round

MAPS: USGS *Blackhawk;* posted on the trail at trail junctures but not at the trailhead; nearby Devil's Lake State Park also has the map in their own park brochure.

WHEELCHAIR ACCESSIBILITY: None

FACILITIES: Restrooms, water pump, picnic tables

CONTACT: dnr.wi.gov/topic/parks/ name/naturalbridge, 608-356-8301

COMMENTS: The hike can be shortened to take in just the bridge. Signs along the path identify medicinal plants used by American Indians. You must pay a state park daily-use fee at the self-service box in the parking lot if you don't have an annual park sticker.

Oak, maple, hickory, and the occasional clump of aspen dominate the forest, and throughout most of the arch portion of the trail, the understory is thin, allowing you to see the rolling earth that escaped the glaciers in this region of Wisconsin, known as the Driftless Zone.

The trail rises into the woods to a trail juncture. Coming from the left is your return route from the loop across the highway; go left here. The climb is moderate, and in many places there are railroad tie–and-earth steps. Another 300 feet up the hill, you may see the old trail that once led to steps up the rocky bluff—ignore it and continue on. At 600 feet from that last juncture, the official path breaks right, heading uphill. This out-and-back trail takes you to the top of the exposed sandstone bluff, where there is a scenic overlook. It's a total of only about 0.2 mile round-trip. Look for shelf fungi on the trees around you and lichens across many of the rock surfaces and tree trunks. A sign on the nature trail educates you on the culinary uses of lichens. At the top, the canopy opens up to sky, and a few cedars occupy the level crown of the bluff, surrounded by small remnants of prairie with Indian grass, little bluestem, and grama grasses. Go to the wooden railing along the right side of the trail and find a bit of a scenic overlook. At the peak of summer, some of the greenery here may be cropping the picture, but you should be able to see the hills beyond and a narrow strip of farmland between them and you. You are at the highest point of this section of the trail.

Back on the main trail, follow as it curves around the top of the ridge and you come to a sign about blackberries and the uses of their leaves. If you come in late summer, you can sample them here for yourself. More railroad-tie steps bring you a bit lower, and you come to an area of slender-trunked maples packed together and struggling to compete with the taller oaks that have taken away most of the sunlight. On your left, pass a wooden

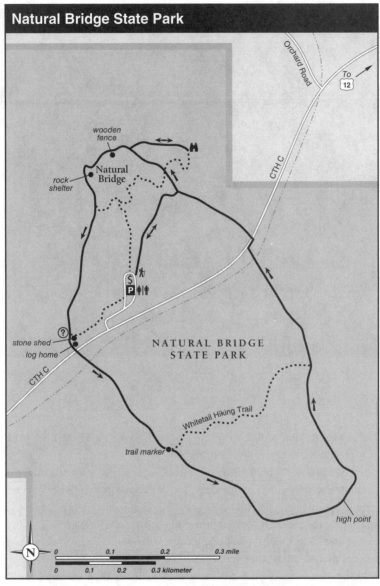

Natural Bridge State Park

- wooden fence
- Natural Bridge
- rock shelter
- stone shed
- log home
- CTH C
- Orchard Road
- To 12
- CTH C
- NATURAL BRIDGE STATE PARK
- Whitetail Hiking Trail
- trail marker
- high point

N

0   0.1   0.2   0.3 mile
0   0.1   0.2   0.3 kilometer

1,200 ft.
1,100 ft.
1,000 ft.
900 ft.
800 ft.
700 ft.
600 ft.

0.5 mi.   1.0 mi.   1.5 mi.   2.0 mi.

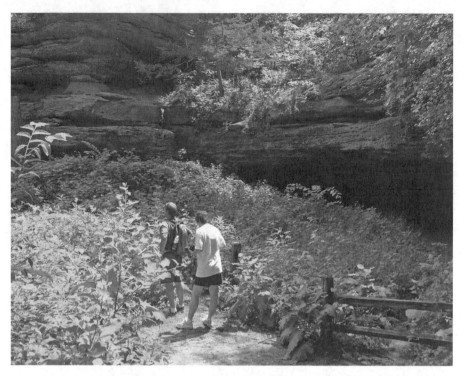

Hikers stop to photograph the rock formation.

fence blocking an old spur trail. This was once a path to the top of the bridge, but entry here is now prohibited to preserve the formation.

Look for witch hazel, which flowers in late fall after all the other trees have dropped leaves. A sign marks its location on the right side of the trail past the wooden fence.

The path descends left with a lot of exposed sandstone. Just a few steps more and you are confronted by the naturally formed bridge of sandstone. The space within the arch is 25 feet across and 15 feet high. A wooden fence keeps visitors from getting too close; in the past, many people carved their names into the soft stone.

The bridge was formed when the mineral deposits holding the sand together dissolved unevenly, and wind and weather erosion left what you see. Look down and to the right to find a large sheltered space in the rock. Excavations of this site in 1967 found charred wood believed to be as old as 12,000 years.

The trail continues on the other side and is shorter and gentler than your first climb. More railroad ties and railings lead to the bottom, where you find another trail map and a sign about poison ivy, hopefully not too late. A trail to the left goes back to the parking lot. In July, look for blackcaps (also known as black raspberries) on this cutoff trail.

Or continue past, staying straight on a wide mowed path through wildflowers in the tall grass to the sides. The trail quickly enters into shade, and the brush closes in around you. Come to a bench on the left. The right side of the trail is another area good for black-caps in early July and some raspberries a few weeks later. This path goes only 900 feet before reentering sunlight via a corridor of sumac. Look for the map board to your right. This mowed area is right on the side of the road, and you see an old log cabin on your right and a smokehouse on your left. Just past the smokehouse is a short wooded trail back to the parking lot.

Cross the road to the hay field on the other side and pick up the trail that crosses straight to the trees 400 feet from the asphalt. The cut-grass path begins a moderate climb into mixed forest. Soon the trail gets a bit more rugged with tree roots; by the time you reach the trail marker for the Whitetail Hiking Trail, it has become a narrow footpath. The trail to the left goes to the edge of the ridge you are climbing and drops down. That segment is difficult and even less developed than the one you are faced with, but it doesn't climb as high.

Keep straight. Underbrush will grab at your ankles, and the shelter of the canopy means dew and previous rains linger longer. Your feet may get wet. The understory rarely rises above the knee, so you can see deep into the woods. You're likely to find far more deer than you are fellow hikers. Be sure to check for deer ticks once you complete the hike.

The trail climbs steeply and starts to head left as it comes upon the highest point of the hike, just less than 0.4 mile from the trail marker. The terrain descends gently at first, and then you come to a patch of ferns and a switchback where the trail goes down even more steeply. The ferns often hide where you are stepping.

There's 0.3 mile of this between the apex and the exit to the hay field. From there, the trail cuts a gentle serpentine path through the field to the road. Cross the road and go right to pick up the trail again. Duck back into some thick woods and go uphill again, crossing a small prairie to arrive at a trail juncture. This is the trail that you came in on; go left and back out to the lot.

Some may prefer to do this trail in reverse, preserving the sandstone bridge and overlook as the big finales.

Nearby Activities

Dr. Evermore (aka Tom Every) is a local artist who has created a menagerie of exotic animals and devices out of scrap metal and odds and ends. His Historical Artistic Memorial Metal Sculpture Park is located on the west side of US 12 just north of CR C and shouldn't be missed.

GPS COORDINATES AND DIRECTIONS

N43° 20' 43.04" W89° 55' 47.49"

Just about 8 miles north of the bridge in Sauk City on US 12, find CR C heading west. Take this 10.9 miles west and find the park entrance on the right side of the road. Follow the short road to the parking lot; the trailhead is on the right behind the toilets; a direct trail is at the north end of the parking lot, if you are going directly to the rock formation.

---

32 Pewit's Nest

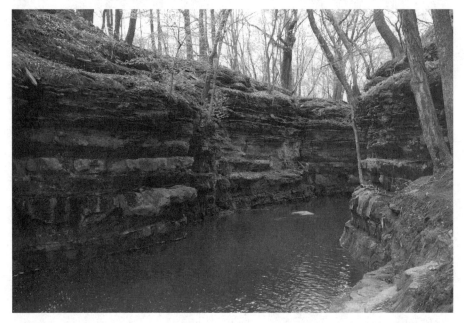

Skillet Creek passes through a gorge.

In Brief

Hike to the mouth of a water-filled gorge, and then climb to the top for views of a creek and a few cascades.

Description

The humble Skillet Creek was once a rush of runoff from the melting glaciers that cut a gorge 30 to 40 feet across—and almost as deep—through fine sandstone that dates back to the Cambrian period, 490 million years ago. Hikers can walk right up to the edge and look down on the gently flowing water that tumbles over three small cataracts. The hike is short but moderately strenuous in a couple of stretches, but most will come here for the view.

Pewit's Nest was given its name by the pioneers who observed a local man who had fashioned a dwelling out of a small cave in the cliffside just above the water. It resembled the nest of a bird called a pewit, also known as a phoebe. The man allegedly used the flowing water of the creek to power lathes. If you stop and ask for directions, be aware that the locals often refer to the area as "Peewee's Nest." It was once just a secret spot known by people from the area, but now the 36 acres form a State Natural Area.

LENGTH & CONFIGURATION: 0.9-mile out-and-back	**DRIVING DISTANCE:** 1.5 miles west from US 12 and County Road W
DIFFICULTY: Moderate with a few difficult parts	**ACCESS:** 6 a.m.–8 p.m. year-round
SCENERY: Towering oaks, wildflowers, flowing water, a gorge	**MAPS:** USGS *North Freedom*
EXPOSURE: Mostly shade	**WHEELCHAIR ACCESSIBILITY:** None
TRAFFIC: Light	**FACILITIES:** None
TRAIL SURFACE: Packed dirt, exposed roots and rocks	**CONTACT:** dnr.wi.gov/topic/lands/natu- ralareas/index.asp?sna=200
HIKING TIME: 0.5 hours for the trail, longer for a swim or exploring the ledges	**COMMENTS:** Leashed dogs allowed. The water is highest in the spring.

The trail cuts into tall grass and passes through a small meadow where crabapples blossom in spring.

The packed-dirt footpath can get quite muddy in the spring or rainy moments. To the left, some of the underlying sandstone layers emerge from the ridge that runs parallel to the trail. Foliage blocks most of this view in the summer, but the trail itself is open to the sky at this point. Another 700 feet from the trailhead, the trees start to close in on the path, and another trail breaks off to the left and rises up into the ridge where the older growth is. This is a short cutoff path and your return trail, so continue straight.

Cross a small clearing and come to a stand of maple saplings with larger trees beyond. Here you find Skillet Creek. There is often a lot of fallen timber here to step over. To your left is the outlet of the gorge. In nice weather, people sometimes swim down here, but low water levels and questionable farm runoff might make that inadvisable.

Go right up to the rising rock at the creek edge and go left along the bottom. The rock will be at your right, and the path gets a little tricky as it climbs, with natural steps formed by rocks and tree roots and strewn with fallen pine needles. If this sort of climb is not your thing, don't worry; you can backtrack the 300 feet to the cutoff point and take the moderate sloping path up.

Climbing here, however, takes you beneath tall pines and through a short, rocky pass until you arrive halfway up the cutoff path. Take this up to the right. Be careful of tree roots here under decaying leaves and needles.

The trail is moderately steep but not treacherous. As you get to the top, the area opens into a wide space beneath the tall oaks and maples and then reaches a fork. Go to the left and head to the ledges overlooking the gorge. The trail continues to the left, but you are going to want to stop here and wander around the ledge to take in the view. The water gurgles softly and foams white below but can get quite a rush on when water is high in the spring or a few hours after a heavy rain. Straight across, you can see more woods that run another 50 feet past the edge before suddenly becoming rolling farmland extending away from this sudden cut in the earth.

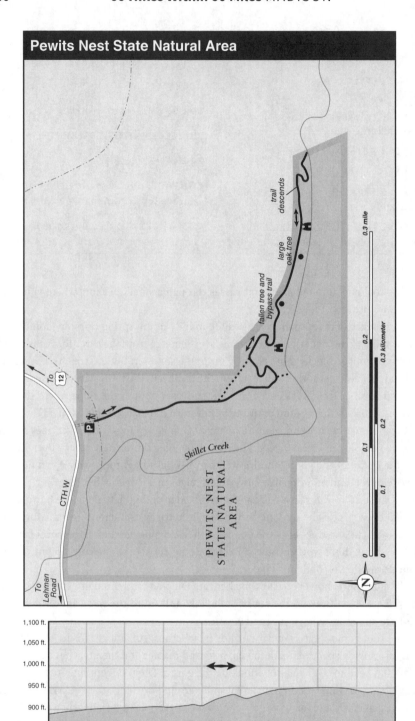

Pewits Nest State Natural Area

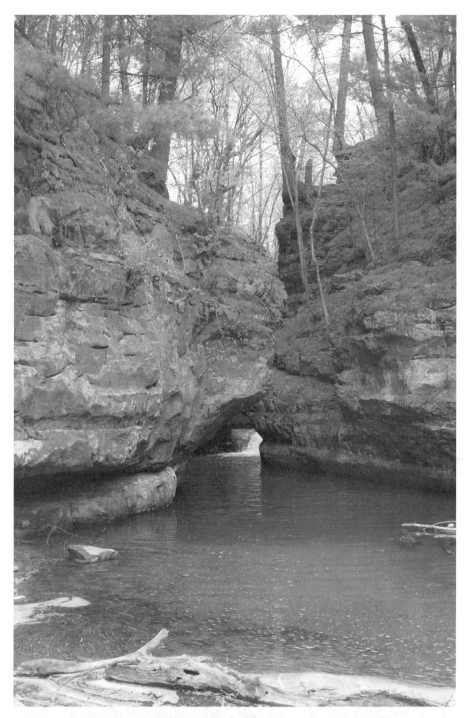

A tiny cascade on Skillet Creek before it flows out from its small canyon

Go right along the upper ledge, which is not quite over the water, until you come to a good place to step down a few feet to the lower ledge, where you can look directly down into the gorge. Take some pictures and take a breather.

Follow the ledge west and see the sandstone supporting the upper levels of the ledge up close at your left. The trail rises up again to the upper ledge just 30 feet later. Watch your step here, especially as you make the few steps up the narrow trail to the packed-dirt trail. Back on the main trail, the edge is not so near and you continue through the forest.

Another 200 feet later, the trail breaks into a short loop to the left that merely bypasses a massive fallen trunk that you have to duck under if you remain on the main trail. Another 200 feet beyond that, it goes both ways around a massive oak trunk that occupies a lookout point on the ledge.

Besides the usual suspects of crows, robins, and blackbirds, kingbirds and the occasional kingfisher will make an appearance here. Squirrels and chipmunks are quite common, and, around dusk, deer may lurk in the nearby cornfields. On some days, the wind will moan through the gorge.

Another 150 feet past the large oak is another good overlook that offers views of the still waters where the creek widens and the silt that lies just below the surface.

The trail heads down a steep and tricky path 100 feet beyond the overlook. This footpath can get slippery in wet seasons. Remember that you'll be climbing back up it to return. At the bottom, find a narrow path over a rock ledge to your right when you are facing the creek. This skirts along the water for about 40 feet to where rock forms a natural dam across the creek. You can step down to the level of the water at the end of this and look down the gorge toward the other end. This isn't a bad place to get your feet wet a little.

Back where you left the trail, continue only another 100 feet to find a farmer's cornfield to your left and the bend in the creek. This is the turnaround point. On your return, stay right; the cutoff trail back at the ledges takes you directly to the main path in the clearing and the parking lot beyond.

In May, the crabapples blossom along the first portion of the trail; in fall, this area is a good place to see the colors.

Nearby Activities

Circus World (866-693-1500) celebrates the history of the American circus with restored train cars and a variety of exhibits, as well as some circus acts during the summer season. It is located in nearby Baraboo at 550 Water St. (WI 113).

GPS COORDINATES AND DIRECTIONS
N43° 27' 9.21" W89° 47' 22.36"

On the south side of Baraboo on US 12 heading north into town, turn left onto CR W and drive 1.5 miles to a small gravel parking area on the left side of the first big curve in the road. The trail starts at the parking lot.

33 Rocky Arbor State Park

A trail through an old river bed

In Brief

Walk along the former bed of the Wisconsin River and see where the glacial runoff and resulting river once dug deep into ancient sandstone, and then climb to the top of the ridge looking over it.

Description

The Wisconsin River once ran through this gorge now rich with a fine mix of forest and wetlands and an assortment of wildflowers. The waterway, which now flows about 1 mile to the east, originally formed at the end of the last Ice Age. As the massive sheets of ice retreated north, a glacial lake formed in the area that is now central Wisconsin, and the outer edges of the ice contained it. When these waters broke through the ice barrier, they rapidly carved paths through the land, exposing and reshaping sandstone laid down during the Cambrian period more than 400 million years ago. Many of the resulting formations that are characteristic of the Wisconsin Dells area are perhaps reminiscent of the Grand Canyon, but, geologically speaking, these were formed "suddenly."

The trailhead is at the far end of the parking lot just past the park office. The trail follows along the edge of the old riverbed and then climbs to the top of the ridge for the return trip. The rock formations along the way make a lovely setting for a short hike, and the wildflowers and wildlife are cause to linger. The mosquitoes, however, enjoy the moist conditions and shelter from the wind, so be sure to prepare for them.

LENGTH & CONFIGURATION: 1.1-mile loop

DIFFICULTY: Moderate to difficult

SCENERY: A gorge, sandstone cliffs and rock formations, mixed forest and wetlands

EXPOSURE: Mostly shaded

TRAFFIC: Light

TRAIL SURFACE: Packed dirt with rocks and tree roots

HIKING TIME: 0.75–1 hour

DRIVING DISTANCE: 0.8 mile southeast

on US 12 from Exit 85 off I-90/94 north of Wisconsin Dells

ACCESS: Memorial Day weekend–Labor Day, 6 a.m.–11 p.m.

MAPS: USGS *Wisconsin Dells North;* map available at park office

WHEELCHAIR ACCESSIBILITY: No

FACILITIES: Campgrounds, restrooms, water, park office, playground

CONTACT: dnr.wi.gov/topic/parks/ name/rockyarbor, 608-254-8001 (summer), 608-254-2333 (off-season)

COMMENTS: Leashed dogs allowed. Be sure to check for ticks after this one.

Just 150 feet from the trailhead, take the short trail to the left and have a look straight down the gorge from an observation deck. Return to the main trail and go left, following the bend of the gorge slightly to the left. Another 150 feet from here, wooden steps go up the cliff face. This is your return route from the upper portion of the trail, but it is also a direct route to the campgrounds up over the ridge and about 0.3 mile away.

Continue past and expect lots of ferns in the understory to the left, while to the right you are looking deep into the past when, during the Cambrian period, this was all sediment at the bottom of a warm sea. The narrow trail is coated with rusty pine needles that seem out of place among the green deciduous trees you see around you. Only by looking straight up do you see the pines that tower above the rest of the treetops and grow farther up the ridge as well.

As you progress, the area to your left becomes marshy, and you see cattails. The trail is narrower still and rather tricky, with rocks and tree roots and a lot of rise and fall. Cross a big, flat piece of sandstone as you pass under a rocky overhang.

In the height of summer, when the ferns are at their largest, there is almost a prehistoric feel to this area.

To your right, look for vertical cracks where tree roots have dug deep into natural fissures in the stone and widened them as they took hold. Some of the trees seem impossibly large to be grasping the rock.

Watch to your right for a sloping gulley that cuts down from the upper level of the ridge to the trail below. Not far past this is a 25-foot-high standing rock to your left, which must have been an island in the middle of the river a long time ago. About 200 feet past this island, look to your right and observe a vertical fissure in the stone.

From here, the trail is wide open to your left. Watch for columbine in the late spring. Flower aficionados will find a few species here that are not found elsewhere in the area.

At just about 0.5 mile into the hike, the trip down the river ends, and you must take the steps up to the right, passing close to moss-covered shelves in the sandstone. Stop

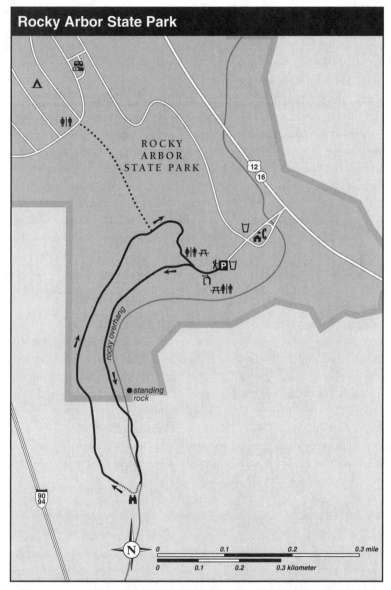

Rocky Arbor State Park

ROCKY
ARBOR
STATE PARK

rocky overhang

● standing
rock

halfway up the staircase to admire the view because, at the top, foliage often prevents a good look. The last portion of the ascent is logs laid in the earth for steps.

When you reach the trail at the top, the highway is just on the other side of the ridge, and traffic noise can be a distraction. The return trail immediately starts to put distance between you and the road hum.

The trail is level through the forest and well shaded by a thick canopy. The trail surface is leaf-covered, and this can hide tree roots, so watch your step. The path begins narrow and widens as you go. About 900 feet down the trail from the top of the steps, look for the channel sloping down to the right, which is the same one you saw from below on the outbound trail. But you won't see that lower trail because it is directly beneath the ridge.

Fine grass growing beneath the trees makes the trail clearer in summer. You come to a juncture where a trail heads left 0.5 mile from the stairs. This takes you to the campgrounds. Go right instead as the trail slopes down gently to a trail marker with an arrow. Here the trail dips again. To the left you can see the lot below in the distance. The path, littered with rust-colored pine needles and showing some shelflike rocks, turns a corner going left down a railroad-tie staircase with a wooden handrail. When it comes around the bend, there's another handrail. Take the steps descending with handrails on both sides to the original trail.

Look up to your left at the bottom and marvel at how little soil lies beneath the trees there. Seeds somehow managed to find a tiny amount of soil in which to sprout atop these rocks, and the root system grew into whatever cracks were present, widening and allowing other soil and nutrients to gather there. The persistence and unlikely strength of these expanding roots eventually widens fissures in the rock, and the most ambitious trees finally destroy their own perches by breaking off the rock. Every once in a while, park managers must take down a tree that is literally teetering on the edge.

Mammals run the gamut here, from woodchucks and squirrels to deer and foxes, and even black bears have been sighted this far south, albeit rarely. It's a short hike so far from Madison, but it's not to be missed.

Nearby Activities

Mirror Lake State Park is just south of here off the same interstate, and, of course, Wisconsin Dells, where the present-day river runs, is a tourist mecca for the state. Take a tour down the river and see the wonderful sandstone formations from aboard an amphibious "duck" at Dells Glacial Park Tours (1550 Wisconsin Dells Parkway, Wisconsin Dells; **dellsducks.com;** 608-254-6080).

GPS COORDINATES AND DIRECTIONS

N43° 38' 24.76" W89° 48' 14.92"

From Exit 85 on I-90/94, take US 12 heading east (actually southeast) 0.8 mile to the park entrance on the right. Pass the office and go straight into the parking lot near the restrooms. The trailhead is at the end of the lot.

34 Rowan Creek Trail

Rowan Creek

In Brief

A stroll along one of the finest trout streams in the state also leads to an island of pine surrounded by wetlands.

Description

One hundred feet into the woods from the parking lot is the first trail juncture, where you will also find a map board. Go left here as the trail goes downhill heading toward Pine Island. The trail surface may show some erosion and some sandy patches. Another 0.1 mile takes you to another juncture. To your left a 0.7-mile lollipop trail takes you out onto Pine Island. The trail to the right is where you continue deeper into the park when you return.

Go left. One hundred feet later, enter cattail marsh and step onto a floating boardwalk. Cross this to the island, where there is a bench alongside the trail to your right. The small island in the middle of the marsh is populated almost entirely by towering pines with a few small oaks scattered along the edges. Just past the bench, cross another smaller boardwalk before you come to the island's loop trail. Go left at the map board.

In the 1930s, this area was converted to pine. The trail follows the western edge of the island, loops around and back, and passes another bench just before completing the 0.5-mile loop. Back at the map board, cross back over to the main trail and go left at that first juncture, continuing east.

LENGTH & CONFIGURATION: 2.8 miles of interconnected loops with an out-and-back segment	**ACCESS:** Year-round
	MAPS: USGS *Poynette;* posted at trail junctures
DIFFICULTY: Easy	**WHEELCHAIR ACCESSIBILITY:** None
SCENERY: Mixed forest, pine forest, wetlands, flowing water	**FACILITIES:** None
EXPOSURE: Mostly shaded	**CONTACT:** dnr.wi.gov/topic/lands/fisheriesareas/2165rowancreek.html
TRAFFIC: Light	
TRAIL SURFACE: Packed dirt, some tree roots and boardwalks	**COMMENTS:** Dogs allowed. Do not confuse this park with another Rowan Creek access point closer to I-39. Cross-country skiing is possible in winter, but trails are not groomed.
HIKING TIME: 1 hour	
DRIVING DISTANCE: 22.8 miles	

This is mixed forest again, mostly hardwoods; at 0.15 mile, you round a point and head right 200 feet to a trail juncture. The straight trail is a cutoff trail that takes you to the return leg of the park loop and back to the parking lot 0.2 mile away. Go left and find water on both sides of the trail. The area to the right is a stagnant pond. Hike 0.1 mile to a bench where the trail goes up over a hump to another juncture and map board. Straight takes you back to the lot. Go left and cross a cattail marsh on a 200-foot boardwalk. You find another bench on the right on the other side. The first trail on your right is the return path off the diminutive Oak Island. Heading left another 75 feet is another map board and the outgoing trail for Oak Island. Save it for your return from the out-and-back trail along the creek. The trail heads downhill to the left, passing another map board.

As signage for the trail points out, this area shows three distinctive habitats. The upland forest is characterized by dry, sandy soil that plays host to oak, hickory, and red cedar, while the moist lowland forest is primarily ash, box elder, elm, and willow. The difference in trees attracts different residents as well; squirrels, turkeys, and grouse tend toward the upland forest, while barred owls, woodcock, and pileated woodpeckers prefer the lowland trees. The third habitat, of course, is wetlands.

Cross a short wooden bridge and then another bridge, following along the main branch of Rowan Creek. You are in the open here with wet prairie to the right. You have another 0.3 mile and one more bridge to cross before the end of the mowed path, where you find the local wastewater treatment plant just beyond the end of the trail. There is parking here on the roadside, as well as a picnic area. An asphalt path leads left to a bridge over the creek and into Pauquette Park in Poynette. If you go just a few paces in that direction, you can see the concrete footings of an old dam. Rowan Creek was once converted to a mill pond. The removal of the dam in 1940 restored the flow and the favorable conditions for trout.

Head back the way you came along the creek. This is one of the best trout streams in the state. Brown trout spawn in November, and springs upstream keep the water temperature

Pine Island

constant in all seasons, making it ideal for the trout eggs to hatch in February. Cross back over the three bridges and come once again to the map board and trail for Oak Island. It is less than 0.1 mile and goes left, returning just a bit farther down your return path.

At that point, go left and return to the 200-foot boardwalk. On the other side, go left at the trail juncture and map board. You have 0.35 mile left to the parking lot. You will pass the cutoff trail coming in from the right at 0.15 mile. Stay left and follow the trail through upland forest until the next juncture and map board, where you will go left 100 feet out to the parking lot.

Nearby Activities

Stop in at the MacKenzie Environmental Center on the east side of Poynette on CR CS/Q. The center is run by the Wisconsin Department of Natural Resources and features prairie restoration with hiking trails, a native animal park with a bison herd, and a museum and interpretive center. Call 608-635-8105 for more information.

GPS COORDINATES AND DIRECTIONS

N43° 22' 51.40" W89° 24' 53.03"

From where it intersects US 151, take I-39 north 20 miles to Exit 115 for County Road J/CS. The exit loops back, so go left (east) on CR CS 2.2 miles to find the park on your left. The trailhead is at the parking lot.

35 Swan Lake State Wildlife Area

Swan Lake is a haven for waterfowl.

In Brief

Explore an overgrown trail along a dike through wetlands to an island of oak savanna surrounded by pockets of marsh and open water. Waterfowl and migratory birds abound.

Description

The difficulty here is not one of inclines but of not always being able to see the trail and, in some cases, having to blaze it yourself through general boundaries. There are a couple of features that will discourage the casual walker: overgrown trails, some with plants with burrs or spines; a potential walk through ankle-deep water for a few feet during wet seasons; and in some cases, lack of any real trail at all. These challenges, however, are part of the attraction. Even the short boardwalk is often camouflaged by all the grasses and wildflowers growing up between the planks, but this gives the hiker a feeling of walking not on water but at least on marshland.

LENGTH & CONFIGURATION: 3.8-mile out-and-back	DRIVING DISTANCE: 34.4 miles north of the I-39 and US 151 juncture
DIFFICULTY: Moderate	ACCESS: 5 a.m.–10 p.m.
SCENERY: Wetlands, oak savanna, open water	MAPS: USGS *Portage;* dnr.state.wi.us
	WHEELCHAIR ACCESSIBILITY: None
EXPOSURE: Mostly sun, with shaded patches	FACILITIES: None
	CONTACT: dnr.wi.gov/topic/lands/wild-lifeareas/swanlake.html
TRAFFIC: Light	COMMENTS: Trail is not marked and in many places is undeveloped and even unclear. Wear long pants and proper footwear. A short, ankle-deep portage across a 20-foot low point in the trail may be necessary. An excellent birding spot.
TRAIL SURFACE: Crushed rock, unmaintained field paths, an overgrown but sturdy boardwalk	
HIKING TIME: 1.5–2 hours	

The Swan Lake Wildlife Area is made up of 1,624 acres, predominantly cattail marshes. This trail follows part of a 1.5-mile dike into the thick of it, then a boardwalk to the "mainland," and then a gravel road out to an island in the middle of it all. You can expect to see sandhill cranes, herons, various species of waterfowl, and other birds, as well as deer, muskrats, and rabbits.

Start from the parking lot and head east 0.1 mile along the edge of CR P, facing traffic. On your return, be sure to pay attention to traffic coming from behind you. Either stay far to the side of the road or cross so that you face traffic for the short distance. The trail begins on the north side of the road behind a large metal gate. Beyond this is a two-tire path through the grassy field following along the line of residences to the right. You will wish you had worn long pants if you come in contact with wild parsley or some of the various thistles, especially when you get to the dike. There are wildflowers through here, goldenrod in particular. Ignore all the spur trails to your right—these merely lead to private backyards.

Locust trees start to take over the terrain as you approach and then enter thick woods and brush at 0.2 mile. The trail is easier to see here, and there are sandy patches. Another 0.2 mile later, pass through the shade of some oaks and then enter the exposed wetlands. To your left is a small pond, and you'll likely find some birds here, perhaps a green heron or some ducks.

The path now follows the dike before you. The trail is not always clear or even there, but the gentle mound of the dike should be apparent. Stay on this and you are fine. You still have a few trees and bushes to your right, but when you pass the last oak tree at about 350 feet along the dike, start watching to your right for the boardwalk, which is only about another 150 feet farther. From that point, if you continue straight, the dike continues another 0.75 mile straight through the marsh, where it angles left for another 0.6 mile, coming out at a parking area at Ontario Street on the north side.

Swan Lake State Wildlife Area

A mushroom appears after a rainy week in August.

The boardwalk is sturdy, but the plant life hides it, so when you look ahead on the path, it always appears as though your path ends about 10 feet in front of you. At the end of this 500-foot walkway, you step down into deep grass and presumably dry, solid earth. Do this carefully because you cannot see where you are stepping. Just a few steps past here is an area of crushed rock and then a gravel road going from right to left. Take a moment to see where you just came out of the grasses, and make a mental note. On your return trip, that boardwalk might not be visible from where you'll be standing.

To your right is a service-vehicle access gate and private property. Go left here along the gravel road and enter oak savanna. You may find some spur trails to the right put in illegally by residents in the neighborhoods east of the area, but stay straight. At 0.4 mile, the trail starts to bend left and exits the woods. A colony of aspen whips line the trail to the left, but to your right, you see straight into the marsh with cattails and some open water. As you continue on the gravel road, the aspens taper off, and there, too, you can see all the way west to where the occasional train passes along the edge of the wildlife area just over a mile to your left.

Another 0.1 mile will bring you to a low point in the road where water flows over the gravel to the other side. After heavy rains or in the spring, this might be 20 feet across but no deeper than your ankles. In dry seasons, it may take just a running jump to get across. If you don't have waterproof footwear, you might take your shoes off and dry off on the other side.

But this is a nice place to take a break anyway. On the other side is what amounts to an island of woodlands in the midst of the wetlands. Oak savanna meets you here, and to your right is a sort of small bay where waterfowl, such as herons and cranes, might take refuge. Birders will want to find a spot among the oaks along the shore to use as a blind.

The path continues on a grassy and perhaps faint vehicle trail into the savanna. Where this trail curves right, you might notice an even fainter trail that continues straight and slightly to the left and takes you out to the edge of the oak savanna along the marsh grasses. This is a nice area to explore as well, offering a view out over the marsh.

The trail described here follows the path to the right. Some may be content to simply explore the area without continuing to the other side of the "island" 0.7 mile away. The park rules allow you to go anywhere. If you continue on the main trail, you cross a small open field roughly 500 feet from your portage. Stay straight and proceed to the other side, where the corridor through the brush bends left and then right again. It starts to leave the oaks, and a thick impenetrable growth of aspen whips shapes the path. Stay left, following the wall of trees and watching for the corridor in front of you when the clearing widens out a bit. You'll soon come to an open field. Stay left, along those trees, and when the aspens taper off, follow the line you are on straight toward another gap in the aspen colony. You will pass a couple of evergreens on your left and walk through a sandy patch. At this point, you have no views of the marsh, and it seems less wetlands than an overgrown sandbar. Continuing down the corridor through the aspens, hike through unmowed terrain. Old tire ruts, invisible in the tall grass, may fill with water or turn an ankle, so be careful.

When you come to a turnaround at the end of the corridor, you see a narrow path through the aspens to the right. Follow it out into the open, where there is a trail cut in the grass, most likely made by local critters trying to get close to the water's edge for a drink. This should bring you all the way to the water. This is the Fox River, flowing into Swan Lake to the east, and your turnaround point.

Nearby Activities

Portage hosts a farmers market from noon to 6 p.m. on Thursdays in season at Commerce Plaza. The 1832 Indian Agency House is on its original site above the Portage Canal, located off WI 33 east of Portage on Agency House Road. It is on the National Register of Historic Places and is open daily for tours May 15–October 15 from 10 a.m. to 4 p.m. Monday–Saturday, and from 11 a.m. to 4 p.m. Sunday. Call 608-742-6362 for more information.

GPS COORDINATES AND DIRECTIONS
N43° 31' 8.42" W89° 24' 16.27"

From its juncture with US 151, take I-39 north 26.5 miles to where it breaks from I-94 and joins WI 78. Continue north on I-39 another 2.4 miles and take WI 33 right into Portage. Go 2 miles to the intersection with US 51 and go right 2.8 miles to County Road P. Go left 0.7 mile. The parking area is on the left. The trailhead is 0.1 mile farther along CR P on the left.

SOUTHWEST

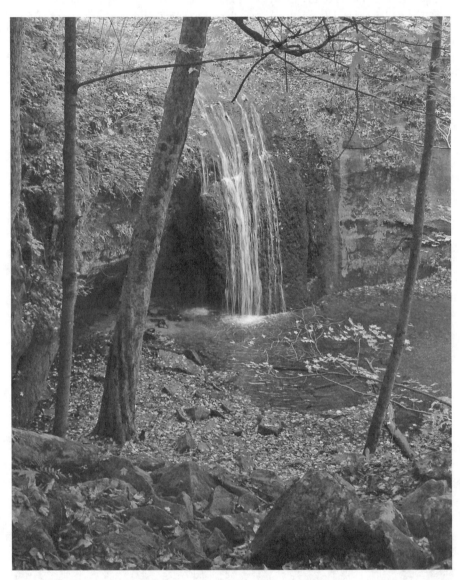

Governor Dodge State Park: Lost Canyon Trail (see page 202)

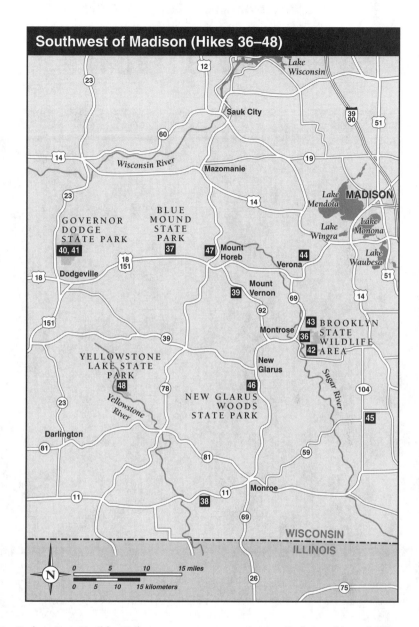

Southwest of Madison (Hikes 36–48)

36 Badger State Trail

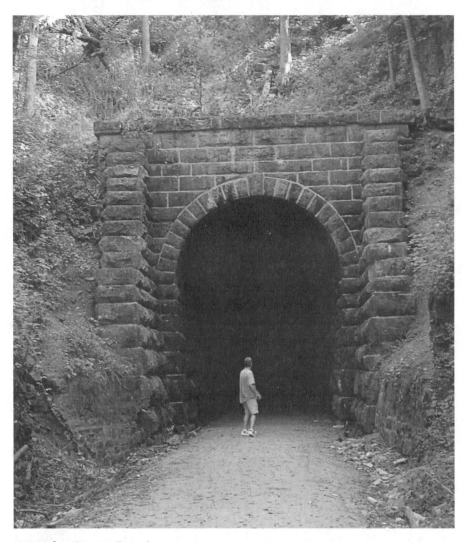

1,200-foot Stewart Tunnel

In Brief

Hike the highlights of southern Wisconsin's latest and arguably greatest rails-to-trails effort as it passes along the line between glaciated and unglaciated terrain, plunges into the dark of a long tunnel, and crosses the Sugar River.

LENGTH & CONFIGURATION: 18-mile out-and-back	**ACCESS:** Year-round
DIFFICULTY: Easy	**MAPS:** USGS *Belleville* and *Monticello*; **badger-trail.com**
SCENERY: Farmland, mixed forest, old train tunnel, river	**WHEELCHAIR ACCESSIBILITY:** Yes
EXPOSURE: Mostly shady	**FACILITIES:** Restrooms at trailheads only; no facilities on the trail
TRAFFIC: Light to moderate	**CONTACT: dnr.wi.gov/topic/parks/ name/badger**
TRAIL SURFACE: Crushed limestone	**COMMENTS:** State trails do not charge fees for hiking, but biking requires a fee ($4 daily, $20 annual). Bring a flashlight for the tunnel and a light jacket if you are susceptible to cold. If you plan to hike the entire length, be sure to bring enough water.
HIKING TIME: 3.5–4 hours (one-way)	
DRIVING DISTANCE: 9 miles south from the exit for WI 69 from US 18/151 near Verona	

Description

Badgers are burrowing creatures, so when European immigrant miners came to south-western Wisconsin—then a territory—for the lead-mining boom in the early 1800s, the seeds were laid for the state's nickname, the Badger State. This hike might make a badger out of you as well because it passes through a 1,200-foot tunnel through an unglaciated hill. The Badger State Trail was inaugurated in July 2007 and is a fantastic conversion of rail bed that connects Madison to the Illinois state border and that state's trail system. If you like the hike, come back with your bike and take it from where it begins in Madison, connected as it is to the Capital City State Trail and Southwest Path.

In Belleville, right across Pearl Street from the parking lot and trailhead is Library Park with picnic tables and a gazebo. If you go west on Main Street (WI 92), you can find several restaurants and bars. The building in the middle of the park is a community center, and, though it has restrooms, it is not always open. The public library has restrooms, or you can seek them out at restaurants on Main Street. There is a place to lock up bikes and a self-pay tube for the trail pass if you choose to ride the trail instead of hiking it. For a good look at the Sugar River, head north on the trail 700 feet (about two blocks from the library) to an old steel railroad bridge.

From the parking lot behind the library at 135 South Vine Street, start south along the trail. Cross Vine Street at an angle and then School Street. From here, the trail is unshaded for 0.7 mile until the first bridge on this segment. On the entire Badger State Trail, there are more than 40 bridges and trestles, in fact, and you cross several of them.

Wetlands ease up around the trail through here; 0.4 mile later, you cross Fahey Road. Another bridge lies 0.6 mile from here and yet another 0.3 mile beyond that. From there, it is only 0.2 mile to County Road W, which heads west 4.5 miles to New Glarus, a small town with a strong Swiss heritage. Before or after your hike, stop in to find Swiss culture, great eats, and the popular New Glarus Brewery.

Badger State Trail

Past CR CC at 0.4 mile, the rail bed was cut into the earth, and the trail becomes a narrow corridor of trees crossing another bridge 0.6 mile later. On the other side of Tunnel Road, find a nice patch of wildflowers before crossing a bridge and entering the channel up to the tunnel. Enjoy walls of rough-cut rock covered with moss on either side of the trail as you approach the dark opening of the Stewart Tunnel, named for the engineer behind the construction of the entire line. The 1,200-foot passageway will be a little chilly even in the heat of summer, and throughout it you can expect to be hit by a few drips in the dark. You can't see the other end of the tunnel due to a bend in its course, so a flashlight is recommended. Part of the tunnel's arch is built of brick; other portions are cut stone, and there is a corrugated metal section as well. About halfway through, you will hear a noise that may disturb you. It is almost as if there is a beating heart there in the earth, a pulsing noise. Fear not: This is merely the cooing of pigeons perched somewhere in the dark. The reverberations of the tunnel have some interesting effects on the sounds. Exit the southern end of the tunnel between stone-block walls.

What lies before you is equally amazing when you think about it. You begin crossing what is essentially a land bridge. You can see that the surrounding terrain slopes down perhaps 100 feet on either side of the path, and treetops rising up from below are at eye level. This rail bed is not the earth and stone removed from the tunnel. In fact, this material had to be hauled in before the equipment to build the tunnel could reach the hill behind you. This must have been some serious manual labor.

At 1.2 miles, you cross Tunnel Road again. You reach Exeter Crossing Road at 0.3 mile and Marshall Bluff Road another 0.7 mile after that. From here, you might call it "the segment of bridges." To the right is more marshland. You cross a bridge in the sun at 0.4 mile, another bridge at 0.8 mile, and *another* bridge 0.4 mile later, until you finally reach the scenic Little Sugar River after 0.3 mile. You might not be surprised, but there is a bridge here.

Look into the woods at eye level to the right of the bridge and forward. The Sugar River Trail passes through the trees there, and you may see other hikers or bikers. Another 800 feet past the bridge, a trestle crosses the trail high above. It is a road to nowhere these days. It also crosses the Sugar River Trail. Two different railroad companies operated the former rails that ran these two trails, and you can see where one side of the trestle is different from the other. Each company built and paid for its half, and then the two portions were connected to make the crossing.

Just past here, a spur trail spans the 30 feet of woods between you and the other trail. From the trestle, it is another 0.3 mile to CR C. At the road, the Sugar River Trail is 100 feet to your right, making the same crossing. Now you cross more wetlands. Weeping willows are common here.

You are 0.6 mile from the end of this hike. Halfway there, a spur trail breaks right and takes you into Monticello. Main Street has a few places to eat. The Dining Room (608-938-2200) is a recommended dinner stop after 5 p.m. Wednesday–Sunday. Stock up for the trail at Gempler's Market, where you can get good sandwiches at the deli.

You can see that the trail continues past your stopping point at CR EE. The Sugar River Trail intersects just 800 feet farther on. The next 12-mile stretch of the Badger State

Trail has no facilities until you reach Monroe. The parking lot shared by both trails is to the right (west) on CR EE, where you will find restrooms, water, and an old depot. This depot doubles as a youth hostel.

Look for wild turkeys and deer along the trail, as well as hawks and songbirds. Black-caps (black raspberries) can be found in many partly shaded places in early July.

Monticello is the best place to start if you want to get on the trail just for the tunnel or combine the Badger and Sugar River trails for an outing. You also have some options for making this hike shorter. There are 3.9 miles between Belleville and the tunnel, but the distance is 4.9 miles if you approach from Monticello. Dropping off a second vehicle at one of the two parking lots is another possibility: Remember, it is 9 miles *one-way*. Crossing roads offer unofficial roadside parking, and the closest cutoffs to the tunnel are the two trail intersections with Tunnel Road. From the south, it's 1.2 miles to the mouth of the tunnel; from the north, it's only 0.3 mile.

Tunnel Road can be reached by driving from New Glarus 4.4 miles on CR W to where CR CC goes south. The northern end of Tunnel Road is 1 mile south on your right. Continuing south on CR CC another 1.5 miles, go right on Exeter Crossing Road to find the southern end of Tunnel Road 1.4 miles on the right.

Nearby Activities

In Belleville, Community Park is a short walk from the library. Check out Lake Belle View, where the main and west branches of the Sugar River come together. In Monticello, you can fish or go kayaking or canoeing in Lake Montesian, which features a wheelchair-accessible pier and a bridge to an island. Nearby community gardens are a nice place to walk as well.

GPS COORDINATES
N42° 51' 30.94" W89° 31' 56.61"

From US 18/151 in Verona, take WI 69 south 9 miles to Belleville. Turn left on East Main Street and take the immediate first right. One block later, at Pearl Street, turn right. The parking lot and trailhead are on your left behind the public library and post office.

37 Blue Mound State Park

A spring in the forest

In Brief

This is the highest point in southern Wisconsin and a brilliant collection of trails, ranging from easy woodland portions to more demanding but scenic detours into uneven terrain along a woodland spring creek. The geology of the park and the views to the faraway horizon are competing stars here.

Description

Check out the observation tower first for an amazing view of sometimes more than 50 miles.

The hike begins to the left of the tower, as you approach it, on Flint Rock Trail. A crushed-rock path with wood-beam steps descends through scattered rocks and boulders and zigzags through mixed forest. Warm, shallow seas that covered this area millions of years ago left evidence in fossils in some of the rocks. A trail sign invites you to look for them. Good luck.

At 0.1 mile, a trail goes left to the campgrounds, but keep going straight. You'll find some interactive interpretive signage, which is great for kids. Many shallow gullies run down the hill from the right and continue down the slope to your left. After rains, this

LENGTH & CONFIGURATION: 5.6-mile loop with many shorter alternatives

DIFFICULTY: Moderate to difficult, but easy with cutoffs

SCENERY: Mixed woods, some prairie, scattered boulders, tiny streams, two scenic overlooks

EXPOSURE: Mostly shaded with some exposed prairie portions

TRAFFIC: Light

TRAIL SURFACE: Crushed rock, packed dirt, loose rock, tree roots

HIKING TIME: 2.5–3 hours

DRIVING DISTANCE: 24.8 miles west from the Beltline Highway (US 12/18) and Verona Road/US 18/151

ACCESS: 6 a.m.–11 p.m. year-round

MAPS: USGS *Blue Mounds;* at visitor center and major trail junctures

WHEELCHAIR ACCESSIBILITY: None

FACILITIES: Restrooms, water, camping, swimming pool, playground, observation towers, showers, pay phones

CONTACT: dnr.wi.gov/topic/parks/ name/bluemound, 608-437-5711

COMMENTS: All vehicles require a park sticker ($7 daily, $25 annual for vehicles with WI plates). Only the mountain-biking trails are open to hiking when the other trails are groomed for skiing. The park participates in the Junior Ranger/Wisconsin Explorer program (see Preface, page 8).

area seems more like a rain forest. Another 0.5 mile brings you to a spur trail and a bench out of the shade.

You cross a lot of culverts, and finally, at 0.4 mile, a small wooden bridge. Just past here is an intersection. Go straight and continue on Flint Rock Trail and the return path for the Willow Springs Trail. Go left here on Willow Springs Trail, where you find a map board, and just beyond that, the Holy Schist Trail going left. This packed-earth trail is narrow and generally for mountain bikers.

The trail continues another 0.4 mile to a wooden bridge and, just past that, a big trail intersection. To the left is a narrow dirt path, which is the Chert Dip bike path. To your right, find a similar path, also for mountain bikes, the Basalt and Pepper Trail. A soft right is the turn of Willow Spring Trail and John Minix Trail. But you go straight and remain on the John Minix Trail heading east. There is a map board to the left.

Erosion on the trail is common, and after big rainstorms, parts of the trail might be washed out.

Cross two footbridges and a large culvert runoff channel before arriving at the next trail intersection 0.2 mile away where the Chert Dip Trail crosses. Another 0.1 mile takes you to a map board and a spur trail to the left out of the park to Mounds Park Road crossing the Chert Dip Trail, which runs parallel to the road at this point.

Continue straight and enter prairie 0.1 mile later. Crossing it, you find more crushed rock on the trail as it passes through a forest with minimal understory but a lot of fallen wood under a tight canopy. It's another 0.1 mile partly in woods, then out into wildflowers and willows before you arrive at the next intersection. Right takes you back toward the center of the park and the east observation tower. Go left here back into woods with brush along the trail. The next 0.2 mile takes you over two bridges and two culverts. After

Blue Mound State Park

Ryan Creek

Ryan Road

Pleasure Valley Hiking Trail

Oxenade Trail

Pleasure Valley Bike Trail

Mounds Road

Mounds Park Road

Walnut Hollow Trail

park entrance

Chert Dip

John Minix Trail

Gneiss & Smooth Trail

Visitor Station

Ridgeview Trail

Pokerville Trail

Military Ridge State Trail

CTH ID

pool

P

P

Basalt & Pepper Trail

East Trail

Spring House

service building

BLUE MOUND STATE PARK

Willow Spring Trail

Observation Tower

Indian Maker Tree Trail

P P P

P P P

Nature Center

Flint Rock Nature Trail

West Observation Tower

P

Holy Schist Trail

0   0.1   0.2   0.3 mile
0   0.1 0.2 0.3 kilometer

N

1,800 ft.
1,700 ft.
1,600 ft.
1,500 ft.
1,400 ft.
1,300 ft.
1,200 ft.

1.0 mi.   2.0 mi.   3.0 mi.   4.0 mi.   5.0 mi.

The view from the observation tower

the second bridge, the Gneiss and Smooth Bike Trail crosses your path, and you come to Mounds Park Road. On the other side, the trail continues as the Pleasure Valley Trail. Find a map board and trails going left and right. Go left on the grassy trail; to the right is a cutoff to skip the Pleasure Valley Hiking Trail, which is challenging, but for me the most beautiful part of the park and a nice place to linger.

The grassy trail heads down through evergreens, exposed. You come to a trail juncture. Going straight is the grassy Pleasure Valley Bike Trail, and, just past this juncture on the left, the mountain bike Overlode Trail goes left. The Pleasure Valley Hiking Trail, however, goes left into the woods, passing a bench on the left and apple trees to the right.

As you head into the cover of the canopy, you come across a creek to the left. Look for a tree with an elbow bend to it near the base. This appears to be an American Indian marker tree or a pretty good coincidence. The spring-fed creek bubbles over rock as it descends, and you get a closer look as the trail goes down a short distance and then switches back left and brings you right to the water. You cross on the rocks, so watch your footing. On the other side, the trail can be hard to see, but it generally follows the creek downhill with the water no farther than 20 to 30 feet to your right. The path goes down over rocks and is very uneven. You come to a large maple, and the trail goes around it to the left, where you see wood logs to the right side of the trail.

The path turns right toward the creek and a sign with a trail arrow. Cross over a 10-foot, 15-inch-wide wood beam over the creek. Straight ahead is a hill. Cross another creek on another wood beam. This stream joins the other off to your left. The trail continues alongside the creek and brings you to six wooden steps. The path goes over some rock behind a large boulder and crosses a short bridge. Go up another short series of steps where the trail resumes, still following the creek.

The trail curls around that hill to your right, comes back to the creek edge, and faces the hill. You see water coming out of the cracks of the wall of rock in front of you. The trail sign says to go left. The stream is to the right now, and the trail is low enough that, in wet seasons, the water might come up over it. Pass over a two-plank boardwalk to the other side of the creek. You must hop some rocks to get across the creek at the next crossing soon after. A crushed-rock path awaits on the opposite bank; follow it away from the creek. But the trail brings you to another creek; cross on a wide wooden bridge with railings and a nice little cascade to the right.

The path goes uphill with creeks to either side as you climb out of a ravine 0.3 mile to the top on a moderate to steep grade, crossing over a giant culvert with wooden railings just before the mountain bike trail crosses. There is a metal gate at the top. At the juncture just after this, go right. Left takes you out of the park to an access road.

Another 200 feet takes you to another juncture. Go left to take the Pleasure Valley Bike Trail, an easy path through open fields with intermittent tree coverage and wildflowers. This will take you 0.3 mile to another juncture and trail map. Go left and cross Mounds Park Road.

On the other side, the trail goes left into the woods. Go left at the next map board and juncture on Walnut Hollow Trail, which takes you on a 0.4-mile half loop through a bit of prairie and then a forest of black walnuts. You come to the other end of the cutoff trail and continue straight. You can see the Military Ridge State Trail to your left, and the trail goes uphill moderately, crossing two bridges and several smaller gullies as it winds its way 0.7 mile to the asphalt connecting trail between Military Ridge and the park. Go right here 0.1 mile to the camping area turnaround. Follow the road straight up to the main park road, where a sign points right to the office. You go left along the right side of the park road. Pass another road to the left to pit toilets and a pay phone. Take the crushed-rock trail here to your right that reads TRAIL TO PICNIC AREA. Cross a wooden bridge and come to a map board. Go left up to the picnic area, passing a storage shed on the left and then crossing a mountain bike trail. From the park road to where you emerge in the picnic area is 0.4 mile. From there, go left, following along the edge of the road until you arrive back at the parking lot and west observation tower. There's water here along the road.

Nearby Activities

The Cave of the Mounds National Natural Landmark, more than 1 million years old, is the most impressive cavern in the Midwest and full of impressive formations. It is open year-round and only minutes from Blue Mound State Park. Call 608-437-3038 or go to **caveofthemounds.org**.

GPS COORDINATES

N43° 01' 35.68" W89° 51' 22.84"

From the Beltline Highway (US 12/14/18), go left 22.7 miles on Verona Road/US 18/151 to County Road F. Go right 0.2 mile and then left on CR ID 0.5 mile. Turn right on Mounds Road and go 0.5 mile to where it turns left and becomes Mounds Park Road. Follow this 0.3 mile straight to the park entrance. Follow the park road 0.6 mile past the visitor center all the way to the picnic area. Follow the one-way road to the right 0.3 mile to the parking area for the West Observation Tower. The trailhead is to the left of the tower.

38 Cadiz Springs State Recreation Area

The dike between the two lakes

In Brief

The dikes through these two lakes are great for birders, and the trails continue beyond, following a spring creek through woodlands and then crossing prairie and farmland.

Description

The trail begins on an asphalt path along the back of a dike between two dam-made lakes—Beckman Lake to the west and the smaller Zander Lake to the east. Early in the morning, you can expect a lot of birds and a few anglers along the dike. Swallows sweep over the grasses and open water, while great blue and green herons hunt along the shoreline. The trail bends left (east); by 0.25 mile, grasses, cattails, and brush close in on the

LENGTH & CONFIGURATION:
4.2-mile figure eight

DIFFICULTY: Easy

SCENERY: Lake, wetlands, mixed forest, prairie

EXPOSURE: Half and half

TRAFFIC: Light

TRAIL SURFACE: Packed dirt, mowed grass

HIKING TIME: 2 hours

DRIVING DISTANCE: 47.7 miles southwest from the Beltline Highway (US 12/18) and Verona Road (US 18/151)

ACCESS: 6 a.m.–11 p.m.

MAPS: USGS *Browntown;* at the park office

WHEELCHAIR ACCESSIBILITY: Along parts of the dike. A toilet and fishing pier/ boat launch are accessible as well.

FACILITIES: Pit toilets, water, play- ground, boat launch, shelter

CONTACT: dnr.wi.gov/topic/parks/ name/cadizsprings, 608-527-2335

COMMENTS: In the past, the park map has been horrifically inaccurate. Changes in mowing patterns may also make this book's map slightly inaccurate in places. Leashed dogs allowed. All vehicles require a state park sticker ($7 daily, $25 annual for vehicles with WI plates).

right side. Two hundred feet later, the dike enters brush completely. The trail is then mowed grass.

At 0.5 mile, find a trail to the right. Just 75 feet past here is a return trail going left, which would take you back around the diminutive Zander Lake via some woods for a very short hike. Take the trail to the right and cross a wooden bridge over the spring creek that feeds the lakes. Be aware: This footbridge can be quite slippery even with a bit of dew. The trail enters thick woods and, 400 feet later, comes to a juncture. Go left here. The right path is the second loop of the figure eight that heads around Beckman Lake.

Another 0.1 mile takes you out to Allen Road. Down the road to your left is a bridge over the creek, but the trail resumes directly across the street. Enter open woods thick to your left, and pass along the edge of a field on your right, which was supposed to be restored to prairie; funding has been delayed.

It's 0.25 mile to the next trail juncture, and halfway there you catch glimpses of the creek through the brush on the left. At the juncture, a trail goes right out to Franklin Road. Stay left and pass through a row of trees and brush to a field on the other side. Another 0.25 mile takes you through the open to the next juncture. Go left. The trail to the right heads out of the park (as any other mowed paths to the right along this section probably would).

Enter the woods, cross over the tiny creek, and then follow the path slightly to the right up into some more trees. Another 0.2 mile takes you into a clearing; 0.15 mile across that clearing, an alternative trail heads left and into the woods opposite. Stay straight back into the forest, passing another trail on the left and continuing 0.15 mile back into the open and the northeastern corner of the park. Go left, with power lines and

Cadiz Springs State Recreation Area

agricultural fields running parallel to the right of the path. Going straight would take you out to Allen Road to bypass the wooded portions of the trail.

Rather, go left at the next juncture as the trail angles away from the park boundary, curving until it is heading due south. Stay straight on this, passing a connecting trail on the left and then following along the edge of the woods to the left as well. The trail turns right and follows between sumacs and a farm field on your right and the woods on the left. Follow it into the woods 0.3 mile from where you left the power lines. Two hundred feet in is the next juncture, and you follow it first to the right and then left as it skirts the woods once more. The trail curves north along the trees and then turns left where you see a path into the woods. Follow this 0.3 mile through mixed forest to reach a clearing and trail juncture with the park maintenance shed on the right. Go right, straight out to Allen Road. Go left on Allen Road, cross Cadiz Springs Road and the bridge to find your return trail on the right—the same trail you emerged from for this half of the park.

Backtrack 0.15 mile to the trail juncture and now head left. The path goes 0.4 mile through woods with open canopy and then emerges next to Beckman Lake, taking you another 1 mile around the edge of the water, passing several benches along the way. At the west end of the lake, the land slopes down to your left and you have a view out over pasture to the farmland and hills beyond. On the north side of the lake, you pass a service road that can take you out to Cadiz Springs Road and across to an optional out-and-back trail into oak forest. Stay along the lake and pass parking, pit toilets, and a playground, as well as a boat launch, before you reach your starting point 0.15 mile later.

Nearby Activities

Whether you are a train enthusiast or not, this little roadside attraction shouldn't be missed: The Toy Train Barn at W9141 Highway 81 in Argyle showcases a real-life engineer's collection of vintage trains running amid several cleverly designed and animated settings. Admission is $5 per adult and $2.50 per child, and it is open year-round 10 a.m.–5 p.m. Call 608-966-1464 or visit **whrc-wi.org/trainbarn.**

GPS COORDINATES
N42° 35' 1.42" W89° 46' 8.99"

From the Beltline Highway (US 12/14/18), go left 7.3 miles on Verona Road/US 18/151 to WI 69. Follow WI 69 south 33.2 miles to Monroe. Go west on WI 11 for 6.1 miles. Turn left on Allen Road, go 0.8 mile to Cadiz Springs Road, and turn right, continuing 0.3 mile to the park entrance on your left. Park in the first lot near the end of the dike, where you will find the trailhead.

39 Donald County Park

A bridge over Deer Creek

In Brief

Two good trout streams cross the prairie, and at the edges of the oak-forest hills, you find apple trees and wildflowers. The trail follows flowing water and then straddles a ridge with rock outcrops.

Description

The Donald/Woodburn family donated the original 105 acres of this park to Dane County. The park has since grown to 480 acres and added a nice picnic area called Pop's Knoll, where a shelter and a couple of fire pits rest amid oak savanna. Deer Creek and Fryes Feeder, two trout streams, run through the park, crossing prairie and farmland, and the wooded portion of the park climbs a nearby ridge.

From the parking lot, go to a service gate in the corner to pick up the trail. To your left is the small hill where the picnic area is. To your right are agricultural fields.

LENGTH & CONFIGURATION: 4.5-mile figure eight	southwest of the Beltline Highway (US 12/18) and Verona Road/US 18/151
DIFFICULTY: Moderate with a few steep areas	**ACCESS:** 5 a.m.–10 p.m.
	MAPS: USGS *Mount Vernon;* at trailhead and junctures
SCENERY: Prairie, flowing water, forest, savanna	**WHEELCHAIR ACCESSIBILITY:** None
EXPOSURE: Half and half	**FACILITIES:** Pit toilets, shelter, picnic tables
TRAFFIC: Light	**CONTACT: countyofdane.com/lwrd/ parks/donald.aspx**
TRAIL SURFACE: Grass, packed dirt	
HIKING TIME: 2 hours	**COMMENTS:** Dogs require a fee ($5 daily, $30 annual) and must be on a leash. There is a self-pay tube in the parking lot.
DRIVING DISTANCE: 13.3 miles	

As you walk down the crushed-stone path, you pass pit toilets and a shelter on your left. Then the trail bends right down the hill. You see woods far across the field in front of you and a bit of oak savanna to your left. A stone path leads to the picnic table and fire pit immediately to your right.

Pass under the Pop's Knoll sign, after which the trail goes left along the fields and at the bottom of the knoll. Look up to your left and see some exposed rock. The mowed area ends here, and you begin down a wide mowed path just 0.1 mile from where you started. Just past here, the trail starts to follow the small trout stream known as Fryes Feeder on your left. Keep following it as the trail bends to the right with its course. Across the stream are a couple of oaks and willows, and the trail bends left again. The stream will take one more big right, and then the trail begins heading toward the woods.

Look for bluebird houses throughout the fields. Fryes Feeder will break left, leaving the trail, and, just 500 feet later, you cross Deer Creek on a footbridge at about the 0.5-mile mark. The trail slopes up to a trail juncture. This is the beginning and endpoint of the loop. There is a map board across the trail to the left, and to your right you find a bench under an enormous willow.

On your right, look for a narrow footpath—hiking only—that follows Deer Creek very closely. The surface is a mix of packed dirt, moss, and grass, and the trail heads west upstream with the creek always just off the path. About 0.2 mile from the bridge, you will pass along sandstone on the left and then cross a footbridge, heading out into the open skies. At the 1.2-mile mark you come to another parking lot, the Deer Creek Fishing Area off Sutter Drive. The hiking trail loops back around to return east, but get out at the parking lot and cross Sutter Drive to continue the second loop of the figure eight.

On the other side of the road, take the branch to the left (your return path is coming toward you), and follow it parallel to the road for 250 feet, where it goes right at a juncture. The trail follows the edge of the woods for 0.2 mile and then enters the trees to begin climbing Hitchcock Ridge.

Donald County Park

This is the hardest part of the hike but also one of the most impressive. Along the ridgetop, you will pass several massive rock outcrops over a quarter-mile stretch. At the end of the ridge, just before the trail takes a left to head south, look for a scenic overview. It deserves a little caution as it steps out on the rock with about a 100-foot drop before you.

Back on the trail, heading south, the trail enters a meadow with a mowed trail around the perimeter. Stay straight until the edge of the park, and then go right (west). This will take you to the opposite corner of the meadow. Continue past, and at the next juncture, take the first right to follow the trail into the woods 400 feet; it comes through a small patch of prairie before heading back under Hitchcock Ridge with the sandstone now visible to your right. The trail passes a large outcrop on your left, and soon you are back on the bridle path, having completed 2.2 miles of the hike so far. The bridle path goes left in a small lollipop that would add about 1.2 miles to your hike. Otherwise, go right here and follow the trail 0.3 mile east to the Sutter Drive parking lot. From the lot, go right on the hiking path. It follows along the bottom of a small ridge for 0.2 mile and then curves right (south) to intersect with the bridle trail again. Cross the bridle trail to continue the hiking-only trail.

On your left is Larson's Pond. A spur trail on the left takes you to a small dock and bench where you can sit and listen to the bullfrogs. Past the pond, the trail turns left (east) and crosses another juncture with the bridle trail. Stay straight and it will pass a bit of pine plantation on the right and head into the woods at about the 3.3-mile mark. The path climbs a small hill and descends 0.3 mile, coming out on the bridle trail about 350 feet west of that first bridge that brought you over Deer Creek. You can go left here for the 0.5-mile return to the parking lot.

This trail system has developed a lot in the last decade, so don't be surprised if some of this changes a bit. Also, there is so much more to hike in this park, including a nice stroll through an apple orchard and along Mount Vernon Creek (which begins just east of the bridge where Deer Creek and Fryes Feeder come together).

Nearby Activities

Put back any calories you may have burned by stopping in at the world-class Candinas Chocolatier in Verona. To find out more about their decadent delights, call 800-845-1554 or visit **candinas.com.** If artisanal cheese is your preference, pick up some locally made varieties at Edelweiss Cheese Shop (204 West Verona Ave., Verona; 608-845-9005; **edelweisscheeseshop.com**).

GPS COORDINATES

N42° 57' 38.02" W89° 40' 30.50"

From the Beltline Highway (US 12/18), go south 7.9 miles on Verona Road/US 8/151 to the exit for County Road G. Go south on CR G 3.5 miles to Messerschmidt Road and go right 1.8 miles to WI 92. Go right just 0.2 mile to the park entrance on the left. At the end of the parking lot to the left is the trailhead at a metal gate.

40 Governor Dodge State Park: Lost Canyon Trail

A spring-fed waterfall

In Brief

Visit a waterfall in a canyon and a cave in the bluffs, and cross hill and vale along Twin Valley Lake before returning through a canyon full of trees and a creek.

Description

The first segment of the path is the only wheelchair-accessible part, but it is recommended for all park visitors. Most everyone stops to walk the asphalt path to see the spring-fed Stephens Falls, which tumbles down into a canyon hidden in the trees.

Just 0.1 mile takes you along a narrow spring creek on the left side of the trail to a juncture. Go straight to see the falls; there is an overlook and a path of rock steps switching back down to the bottom of the canyon. Return to the trail juncture and begin the Lost Canyon Trail, crossing the bridge and passing the Spring House, where the waters emerge from the earth. Go uphill on grass, pass through a stand of tall pine, and enter prairie. Just outside the woods, this prairie portion of the trail hits a T. Go left. The right trail is the return of 2.5-mile Gold Mine Trail.

Pass through prairie, crossing the park road at 0.3 mile and arriving at a juncture 0.1 mile later. A trail to the left connects to the equestrian trail. Go right on a two-tire path with scant shade through oak, walnut, basswood, and hickory. At 0.4 mile, you pass the Gold Mine Trail on the right for an optional return to the area of the falls. Stay straight;

LENGTH & CONFIGURATION:
8.8-mile loop

DIFFICULTY: Moderate

SCENERY: Flowing water, waterfall, cave, hardwood forest, rock formations, lake

EXPOSURE: Half and half

TRAFFIC: Light

TRAIL SURFACE: Packed dirt, mowed grass, crushed rock with a short asphalt segment

HIKING TIME: 3 hours

DRIVING DISTANCE: 44 miles from the West Beltline Highway (US 12/18) and Verona Road/US 18/151

ACCESS: 6 a.m.–11 p.m. year-round

MAPS: USGS *Pleasant Ridge;* at the park office

WHEELCHAIR ACCESSIBILITY:
0.25-mile asphalt trail to Stephens Falls overlook

FACILITIES: Restrooms, water, picnic tables, boat landing, concessions, campgrounds

CONTACT: dnr.wi.gov/topic/parks/ name/govdodge, 608-935-2315

COMMENTS: Portions of the trail are shared equestrian trails. All vehicles require a park sticker ($7 daily, $25 annual for vehicles with WI plates). Pets must be leashed except in designated pet swim areas. The park participates in the Junior Ranger/Wisconsin Explorer program (see Preface, page 8); activity books are available in the park office. Hiking is not allowed in winter when this trail is groomed for skiing. Consider White Oak Trail or consult the park office at 608-935-2315 for other options.

another 0.6 mile takes you to a spur on the right out to the equestrian trails. The Lost Canyon Trail goes right, passing through sumac. To your right is a fine view of the prairie as you head downhill. Pass a bench as the trail curves left around the edge of forest and into trees at 0.15 mile. The trail becomes mostly shaded through the woods as you continue 0.65 mile to the next horse trail juncture, passing a small creek at 0.35 mile.

Across the wide grassy horse path, stay straight, heading uphill into a loop that rounds the large bluff before you. At 0.1 mile, an optional cutoff trail to the right skips the loop. Go straight another 0.5 mile, passing close to the shoreline of Twin Valley Lake before arriving at a spur trail to the right. This heads up the ridge 0.1 mile to the crown, where you can find a cave. Follow the signs, and the trail climbs to the top; go right and back down to the right a bit in front of the rocky bluff face to find it.

Back on the main trail, descend to the right, pass cattails along the shore, and reach the cutoff trail at 0.4 mile. Go left, heading into woods to another trail juncture. This is the horse trail coming in from the right, so stay left; 0.1 mile later, enter prairie. The lake is to the left; follow a grassy trail amid wildflowers. Go left at 0.1 mile at the next juncture and continue through prairie with your best view of the lake. You can see the bluffs you just visited across water.

The trail goes back into woods for 0.2 mile, following the edge of a gully, with exposed rocks to your right and sand on the trail. The trail crosses left over a culvert and then heads back into the open for another 0.4 mile of prairie and brush. Cross a culvert into the woods and continue with shade for 0.3 mile. You start to hear Mill Creek flowing to your left in the open. Another 0.2 mile brings you to the concessions and a parking lot.

Governor Dodge State Park: Lost Canyon Trail

There are toilets and water here. A trail to your left will connect to the Military Ridge State Trail. Go right along the edge of the parking lot to the next corner. The trail heads up into the woods and bends right as it climbs. A line of rocks separates the trail from another trail to the amphitheater area.

From the lot, it is 0.1 mile to the amphitheater entrance. Continue past on asphalt, passing a wheelchair-accessible parking spot. An arrow looks like it leads you to the right into the woods, but it is only to indicate that you should not follow the curve of the asphalt but stay straight on the grassy trail that leads you through prairie and an aspen colony 0.3 mile to the woods again.

Just inside the trees, come to a poorly marked intersection. Left takes you back to the beach area. Go right 0.1 mile to a four-way intersection and go left toward the park road, crossing through prairie. Straight takes you into Twin Valley Campground; the trail to the right is the horse path. At the park road, a two-tire path descends through spruces 0.1 mile to another meeting of the equestrian path. Go right here and head through prairie for the next 0.5 mile, briefly passing through a grove of locust trees and finally arriving at the horse path going left to right. Go straight across and 50 feet to another juncture. Lost Canyon Trail goes left and follows along the edge of the Cox Hollow Campground. It gradually slopes into the canyon, switches back at 0.3 mile, and takes you another 0.2 mile to a creek running through a culvert.

Now you start to see some mammoth rock outcroppings to the left. Water flows toward you on the right, and at 0.5 mile from the culvert, you cross a wide wooden bridge over the creek. Two more bridges await before the next trail juncture at 0.15 mile.

The path to the right follows the creek 0.2 mile to Stephens Falls. This is a good cut-off option. Otherwise, continue left, crossing a footbridge and following another smaller creek coming down the hill in front of you, until you arrive at the park road 0.3 mile later.

Go right here along the road's edge 200 feet as the trail cuts back into woods briefly and then out into prairie for the home stretch. Hike 0.3 mile to the asphalt trail and go left back out to the parking lot.

Nearby Activities

The Frank Lloyd Wright Visitor Center and Taliesin Home, at WI 23 and County Road C in Spring Green, is open May–October. This National Historic Landmark offers guided tours. Call 608-588-7900 or go to **taliesinpreservation.org.**

GPS COORDINATES
N43° 01' 37.53" W90° 07' 52.95"

From the West Beltline Highway (US 12/14), go southwest 37.4 miles on Verona Road/US 18/151. At Exit 47 for Dodgeville, take US 18 west for 1.9 miles and then turn right on Bequette Street/WI 23 for 3.3 miles to the park entrance on the right. Take the park road 0.25 mile past the office and go straight at the first intersection, following the road 0.8 mile to the roadside parking lot at the trailhead to Stephens Falls.

41 Governor Dodge State Park: White Oak Trail

Cox Hollow Lake

In Brief

Hike the shores and climb the rocky bluffs overlooking Cox Hollow Lake. Then visit a prehistoric rock shelter.

Description

From the trailhead, pass to the right of the concessions stand and a trail kiosk. Go straight ahead downhill just 400 feet to where the water flows over the dam to the right. Cross a wide wooden bridge to see the water tumbling over rocks to your left. Either follow the asphalt path straight across or, better yet, climb the earthen dam to your right and follow along the top of it as it skirts Cox Hollow Lake. There are no natural lakes in the southeastern corner of the state, known as the Driftless Zone; the glaciers didn't arrive here to leave damming deposits in river valleys. To the right, you can see rocky cliffs on the other side of the lake. That is where you are headed.

It's 0.1 mile across the dam and into the woods. To your left is the return trail for the 3.3-mile Mill Creek Trail. Several paces beyond this, the trail forks. Up to the left on asphalt is the start of Mill Creek Trail. Go right on a packed-dirt and crushed-rock footpath, which is the White Oak Trail. Only 250 feet along is the juncture with Lakeview

LENGTH & CONFIGURATION:
4.3-mile loop

DIFFICULTY: Moderate

SCENERY: Mixed forest, cliffs, exposed rock, lake, wetlands, rock shelter

EXPOSURE: Mostly shaded

TRAFFIC: Light

TRAIL SURFACE: Mostly packed dirt, rocks and roots, with some grass, cedar chip, crushed rock, and asphalt

HIKING TIME: 1.5 hours

DRIVING DISTANCE: 45.8 miles from the West Beltline Highway (US 12/18) and Verona Road (US 18/151)

ACCESS: 6 a.m.–11 p.m. year-round

MAPS: USGS *Pleasant Ridge;* at the park office

WHEELCHAIR ACCESSIBILITY: None

FACILITIES: Restrooms, water, picnic tables, boat landing, concessions, campgrounds

CONTACT: dnr.wi.gov/topic/parks/ name/govdodge, 608-935-2315

COMMENTS: A 1-mile segment of this trail is a self-guided nature trail. Pets must be leashed, except in designated pet swim areas, and are not allowed on the Pine Cliff Nature Trail segment. All vehicles require a park sticker ($7 daily, $25 annual for vehicles with WI plates). The park participates in the Junior Ranger/Wisconsin Explorer program (see Preface, page 8); activity books are available in the park office.

Trail. If you go left, this loop adds another mile to your hike and rejoins this trail just 0.15 mile farther along. White Oak continues along the lakeshore, passes the Lakeview return trail, and goes right and across a culvert before it heads back around a finger of the lake to your right. The trail becomes narrower as it heads into thicker forest and gradually turns more and more rugged with roots, rocks, and uneven surfaces.

The trail goes around a rocky outcropping to the left and starts to curl up left over tree-root steps through forest dominated by native pine. From the juncture to the top is 0.3 mile where the trail may be difficult to discern in the carpet of pine needles. Watch for it to the left where it heads back down the rocky bluff. This area at the top is Raccoon Point, and you can follow it out to the end with a drop-off to either side. Return along the opposite side to come to the trail as it continues past the point.

The path goes to the right and down with a lot of tree roots and loose sandstone. It winds around trunks and boulders 0.2 mile to the bottom, where it crosses a small wooden footbridge over a creek. The trail bends left and follows the creek, curves when it reaches the lake, and heads uphill to a smaller cliff. You are now getting looks into the marshy area at this corner of the lake, which is great for spotting waterfowl.

At 0.3 mile from the bridge, the trail comes out to an access road and a map board. To the left is the park's horse trail. Go right to continue on White Oak Trail. This area can get a little soggy in spring or during rainy periods, but the grass keeps it from getting too muddy. There is a bench here for a quiet spot to observe the marshy area. On the other side of this open stretch, the trail curves right, passing over a muddy spot with a few stepping-stones or branches in wet seasons. The path widens and becomes grassy with sandy patches.

Governor Dodge State Park: White Oak Trail

At 0.2 mile from the bench, the trail forks. You can stay left for White Oak, but it's better to take Pine Cliff Trail to the right. The 1-mile, self-guided nature trail offers educational signage as it climbs a bluff on a narrow footpath. It starts along the lake's edge, then climbs left moderately with some log and dirt steps. At the top, go right at the map board and there is a 20-foot-high outcropping of rock. There are no easy steps, but it is climbable to the next surface, which is a flat area that offers various scenic overlooks of the lake at the end of the bluff.

Return from the point, climb back down the rocks, and follow the spine of the ridge, passing your arrival trail. The trail goes 0.5 mile back to White Oak Trail, where you go right and down into a hollow, coming to a bridge over a ravine of water-smoothed stone. Across the bridge, stairs go down the other side of the ravine. From the bottom of the steps, it's 0.3 mile to a parking area. Cross a narrow footbridge and pass a lot of exposed rock as you follow a creek on your right. You go over the creek as you enter the parking lot. There is a kiosk and restrooms to the left and a water pump in season.

Go right out to the main park road. This is Enee Point rising above you ahead to the right. Straight across is Box Canyon. There are no "official" trails up to the point, but the hike is permissible for those looking for a short but challenging climb with a view at the end.

Go right on the park road and follow it back to where you started. Alternatively, you could double back the way you came on White Oak Trail. Along the park road at 0.7 mile, you come to Deer Cove Picnic Area on your left just after a boat landing area on your right. Look for a spur trail to the left when you are facing Deer Cove. A 350-foot trail leads up to a rock shelter that has evidence of being occupied by Paleo Indians between 7000 and 6000 B.C., clearly the oldest of the campsites in the park. Back on the road, it's another 0.2 mile to the road to the modern campgrounds on the left and then another 0.1 mile to the parking lot and the trailhead.

Nearby Activities

The House on the Rock (5754 WI 23, Spring Green; 608-935-3639; **thehouseontherock. com**) is an odd attraction, containing rooms full of exotic collections and the world's largest carousel. Truly, it must be seen to be believed.

GPS COORDINATES
N43° 00' 53.02" W90° 06' 18.67"

From the West Beltline Highway (US 12/14), go southwest 37.4 miles on Verona Road/US 18/151. At Exit 47 for Dodgeville, take US 18 west for 1.9 miles, and then turn right on Bequette Street/WI 23. Go 3.3 miles to the park entrance on the right. Take the park road 0.25 mile past the office and turn right at the first intersection; go 2.5 miles to the parking lot. The trailhead is to the right of the concessions building.

42 Ice Age Trail: Brooklyn Wildlife Segment

Descending into prairie from a forested ridge

In Brief

Get some up-close views of sandstone formations in the forest, and take in vistas over the prairies, on this rugged segment of the national trail.

Description

Many of the glacial formations in the area are said to have been left when the last of the most recent glaciers retreated north 10,000 to 20,000 years ago. The moraines on this segment of the trail are believed to be from glaciers of an earlier advance more than 60,000 years ago.

The trailhead is in the gravel parking lot at the southern end of the segment. A map is posted there. The path heads north 0.2 mile across open prairie and follows various trees along the way marked with yellow painted squares, which are useful in winter. The trail is maintained, but often the grass gets a little long. It is exposed here. Entering the

LENGTH & CONFIGURATION: 6.8-mile out-and-back	**ACCESS:** Year-round
DIFFICULTY: Moderate to difficult	**MAPS:** USGS *Attica* and *Oregon*; posted maps at trailheads
SCENERY: Prairie, mixed forest, glacial moraines	**WHEELCHAIR ACCESSIBILITY:** None
EXPOSURE: Some shade, a lot of sun	**FACILITIES:** A single water pump on the trail
TRAFFIC: Light	
TRAIL SURFACE: Narrow packed-dirt footpaths with roots and rocks; grassy paths	**CONTACT: iceagetrail.org,** 800-227-0046
HIKING TIME: 3.5 hours	**COMMENTS:** Some portions of the wooded areas are overgrown with snagging plants, such as raspberries and similar thorny tendrils. Long pants are advised. Leashed dogs allowed.
DRIVING DISTANCE: 10.4 miles west from US 14 and WI 92 south of Madison	

woods, the trail begins sloping gently downhill and becomes packed dirt with a covering of dead leaves.

Just 0.4 mile later, you enter a clearing. Fire lanes go off to either side but are overgrown though still passable for further exploration. There is a plethora of wildflowers through here. The trail starts uphill soon after and passes through some small oaks, coming to the crest of the hill before sloping down, partially shaded by the canopy.

The trail veers left, but go straight according to the yellow blaze on a tree. There are sandy patches here along the trail. As you come over the crest 150 feet later, you have a few steps of tree roots and earth.

There are plenty of tree roots under the dead leaves, so mind your footing. You'll go over another hilltop 400 feet later and then follow the trail down a slope along pine trees that have carpeted the surface with needles.

At the bottom of the slope, the path might be difficult to see if no one's been through in a while, but bear straight ahead as it heads back into woods. The trail curves and comes up to a small pine grove with a trail marker and map showing where you are. Follow the yellow arrow to the right. The path to the left takes you out to an alternate parking lot.

Continuing along the trail, look left and see some of the exposed sandstone from the glaciers' cutting work. The trail is downhill and mostly sand with scattered rocks and tree roots for about 700 feet. Above your head on both sides is exposed rock.

Head into a small clearing. One trail goes left and another goes straight. The official trail is left and takes you higher up to a water pump just before the path heads into the woods. The trail to the right sidesteps the woods and can be an alternate return through the prairie on your way back to the trailhead.

The next 0.6 mile is through forest. At the highest points, the trail looks down the rocks to the left and the slope to the right. You can see quite far down the hill through the

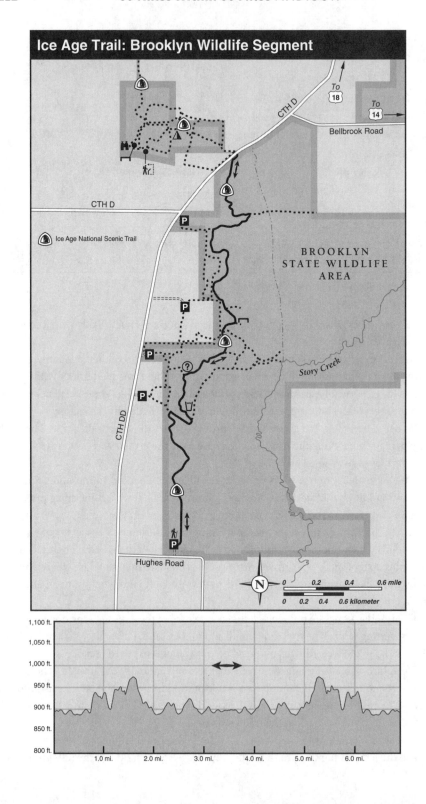

Ice Age Trail: Brooklyn Wildlife Segment

To 18

To 14

CTH D

Bellbrook Road

CTH D

Ice Age National Scenic Trail

BROOKLYN
STATE WILDLIFE
AREA

CTH DD

Story Creek

Hughes Road

N

| 0 | 0.2 | 0.4 | 0.6 mile |
| 0 | 0.2 | 0.4 | 0.6 kilometer |

1,100 ft.
1,050 ft.
1,000 ft.
950 ft.
900 ft.
850 ft.
800 ft.

1.0 mi.   2.0 mi.   3.0 mi.   4.0 mi.   5.0 mi.   6.0 mi.

Wild blackcaps and raspberries are abundant along the trail.

forest and gain an appreciation for the rise and fall of the land if the trail hasn't already made that pretty clear. From here, you will descend almost 100 feet in 2,100 feet. To the left, the land slips into a groove between two hills. The trail dips into this and crosses, and when you climb to the opposite side, you find a trail map. To the left is the trail to the parking lot at County Road DD. Go right and enter a clearing. In summer, you can find raspberries and their thorny shoots. The thorns, combined with the mosquitoes and ticks, make long pants a good idea in most weather.

Head to the bottom of the next gully and bear right. Follow along the bottom of the gully, with a ridge rising up on either side of you. Foliage blocks views of exposed rock, except in early spring and late fall. Look to the right almost 1,000 feet from the map board and there is a Department of Natural Resources (DNR) trail. Go left up the hill, staying with the yellow arrows as the trail passes through more wild berries before it widens and becomes grassy as it comes into a clearing. At the next intersection, go left. The trail to the right returns through the prairie. Stop for a nice view of the valley below this point known as Crane Overlook.

From here, the trail descends to the left through a grassy meadow. Land rolls away, with clumps of forest dotting the landscape. Pass a trail post, and the land drops even farther. As the trail levels off a bit, stay straight along the top of the ridge, keeping the view on either side. To the left, see a traditional red barn. Lichen-covered rocks peek through the prairie grass as you come to a bench 30 feet left of the trail. Pass a row of oak and pine to see across the prairie to the woods beyond. Find another trail marker just before the trail descends through grass and wildflowers. Tire ruts from park vehicles may lurk below the grass on the trail, so be careful.

You come to the woods. This next 0.6 mile is on a narrow trail and can be the worst of the snagging plant life, so be prepared. Raspberries are a midsummer reward. When you exit the trees, you come to a trail marker that leads you right, where you'll find a map board. The trail left heads out to a parking lot.

Now the trail is open, with tall grass and trees not far off to either side. As you pass another trail marker, the prairie opens up and your view stretches for a couple of miles. A double tire lane heads into the field and takes you 0.2 mile to a rocky platform with sandy patches overlooking a berry patch and the prairie beyond.

The trail might be hard to follow over this surface, but as you come over the rise, just keep straight, and you should see the trail marker at the edge of the forest. Go left here 500 feet along the edge of the forest, but don't expect any shade. The trail heads right into a mix of forest and grassy patches for another 0.2 mile before you see signs of civilization again. Pass a trail marker on your right and head across an open meadow with raspberries on both sides. Head for the clump of woods on the other side and pass along the left side of them. The trail enters shade there and curves with the edge of the trees until it meets CR D.

It's up to you where you want to end this hike: As indicated, this is the turnaround point, but you can continue across the highway to connect to the Montrose Segment, just a half mile up the hill into the woods. A prairie loop and scenic overlook to the west can be found here, as well as a Dispersed Camping Area for thru-hikers. Another alternative is to leave off at that last parking lot before you reach CR D. Unfortunately, there is no designated parking lot at CR D.

Nearby Activities

Lake Belle View in Community Park in nearby Belleville to the west is a pleasant spot for a posthike picnic.

GPS COORDINATES

N42° 50' 35.24" W89° 29' 57.12"

From Madison, head south on US 14 (Park Street) and continue 13.7 miles from where it passes under the Beltline Highway (US 12/18). Turn right (west) on WI 92 and follow it 9.2 miles west to Hughes Road. Go north (right) 1.2 miles, following the road as it turns left. The parking lot is on your right. The trailhead is at the parking lot.

43 Ice Age Trail: Montrose Segment

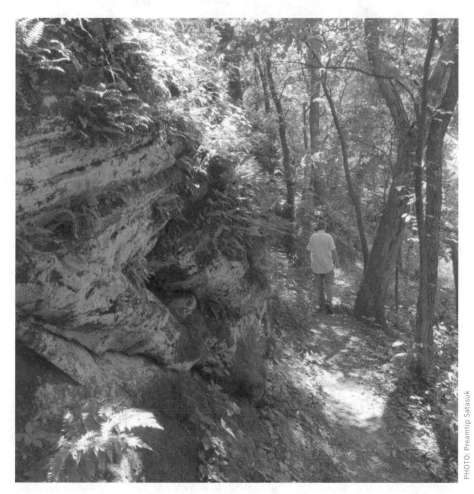

PHOTO: Preamtip Satasuk

The Ice Age Trail passes rock outcrops on the Montrose Segment.

In Brief

A lovely Ice Age Trail segment, Montrose passes along sandstone outcrops along a long ridge, rising to a beautiful bluff-top overlook and ending with a turn around prairie restoration before coming back the way you came.

LENGTH & CONFIGURATION:
4.6 miles; lollipop or optional thru-hike

DIFFICULTY: Moderate

SCENERY: Hardwood forest, prairie, farm fields, bluff overlooks

EXPOSURE: Mixed

TRAFFIC: Light

TRAIL SURFACE: Packed dirt, tree roots, mowed grass

HIKING TIME: 2 hours

DRIVING DISTANCE: 19.8 miles from the juncture of US 14 and US 12/18

ACCESS: Year-round

MAPS: USGS *Verona; Ice Age Trail Atlas;* at trailhead

WHEELCHAIR ACCESSIBILITY: None

FACILITIES: Possible portable toilet in season

CONTACT: iceagetrail.org, 800-227-0046

COMMENTS: Leashed dogs allowed. Dispersed camping permitted in designated area for thru-hikers only.

Description

From the segment that passes along the rail-to-trail Badger State Trail, the Ice Age Trail heads east to hit Piller Road before coming south to the trailhead here. Before being developed, the southern portion of this trail was merely the end loop of the Brooklyn Wildlife Segment, which, at the time, still needed to be connected to the larger trail. Start your hike here from the lot by heading south along the edge of farmland. After 0.1 mile, the packed-dirt path heads into the forest. It takes a turn to the west and follows the edge of a ridge with some switchbacks to gain elevation.

Nearby is a lot of dairy farming, so you might occasionally get a whiff of Wisconsin's dairy air. As you follow the trail, you'll notice a lot of sandstone rock outcrops up the ridge to your left. Come around another rock outcrop at about a quarter mile and the trail takes a turn to the south as it comes around the ridge. Just before the half-mile mark, the trail heads east through open meadow being restored to prairie. Head straight through to a row of trees and brush that creates a border between this and the next section of prairie. Beyond the trees, the path curves to the west and slopes gently before slipping back into the woods at 0.8 mile.

Now begins a slow descent in an easterly direction with a ravine on your right. The trail comes around the ravine's eastern end and heads south. At 1.2 miles, the trail comes out of the forest and crosses agricultural fields with views of the rolling farmland to the right. Take care through here, as the grassy cover can hide large stones and ankle-turning potholes in the trail surface.

The trail continues south, skirting the edge of the trees on your left and even passing through them briefly. Ahead is a line of trees sticking out west from the woods like a fence line. The trail goes left into the forest just before that at 1.4 miles. Many old oaks tower above the trail, which climbs again to follow the edge of the ridge. At the top, you will come into an open meadow with a mowed trail around its perimeter. A blue-blazed trail connects to that loop. But continue and the trail comes to another prairie just outside the

Ice Age Trail: Montrose Segment

Piller Road

Frenchtown Road

To 14

To 69

rock outcroppings

BROOKLYN STATE WILDLIFE AREA

To 18

CTH D

Ice Age National Scenic Trail

N

0   0.1   0.2   0.3 mile
0   0.1   0.2   0.3 kilometer

trees to your left off a short spur trail. Continue amid the trees, and the path bends away from those fields a bit until you arrive at an open area at the top of the bluff. The view here is of a glacial outwash plain. Directly before you is another prairie restoration in progress: Young's Prairie.

The trail continues past here and comes out into that open field you've been seeing through the trees. This is Young's Goat Prairie and Oak Savanna Restoration Project. You will step across the mowed outer loop and follow the Ice Age Trail right through its center to the woods near the opposite corner. You can see a post marked yellow to reassure you that this is still the trail. On the other side of the field, you will find the sign for the Dispersed Area Camping at the end of a blue-blazed trail about 500 feet long. You will also see the yellow-marked connector trail, which could lead you about 0.5 mile through the forest to CR D, where the Brooklyn Wildlife Segment connects from the other side of the road. However, there is no parking at that crossing.

Instead, go left and follow the mowed trail in a long loop around the field until it brings you back to where you entered it on the Ice Age Trail. From here, you can backtrack all the way back to the parking lot. Another section of prairie restoration is to the east of this loop and has similar widely mowed paths around it if you are inclined to explore there.

Nearby Activities

For a much longer Ice Age Trail thru-hike, start at the connecting Brooklyn Wildlife Segment to the south and follow through Montrose, a portion of the Badger State Trail, and the Verona Segment all the way to Madison.

GPS COORDINATES

N42° 53' 31.7" W89° 30' 29.2"

On US 14 heading south from the Beltline Highway (US 12/18), go 10.6 miles and turn left (west) on CR A. Stay on CR A for 8.8 miles until you reach Frenchtown Road in the middle of a curve. Take the slight right off CR A and continue 1.5 miles to the parking lot on the left side of the road. The trailhead is at the end of the lot.

44 Ice Age Trail: Verona Segment

In Brief

Climb through prairie restoration overlooking Verona, cross through suburbia in the shelter of woods, and follow a creek on this portion of the Ice Age Scenic Trail, which ends in a popular dog park.

Description

From the parking lot, there is a wooden sign over the trailhead close to the road. This is not to be confused with a paved multiuse trail that also departs from this lot and runs parallel to the Ice Age Trail, joining it briefly inside Verona. The trail starts out going west along the edge of CR PD for 0.1 mile, then angles left to cut through restored prairie resplendent with wildflowers. A mowed path circles the prairie section and connects to the bike path. Cross the prairie for 0.2 mile, and then you will cross that outside mowed loop just as you enter the trees under thick canopy on a path that slopes gently downhill. The packed-dirt footpath is narrow and uneven. At the peak of summer, thorny raspberry bushes may run rampant, and you are going to want to wear pants through here.

After another 0.2 mile, you come back out of the woods at Reddan Soccer Park; you will find various signs with information about the trail, ecology, and geological history. Continue on the trail 0.5 mile through prairie rich with native wildflowers and grasses. Pass a spur trail on the right to the trailhead in Reddan Soccer Fields, where you find parking, water, and restrooms. Past this, cross a service road, and then come to Cross Country Road. Go right along the wooden fence by the soccer field until you come to an opening marked with a trail sign. Cross the street directly and find a similar gate through the wire fence there. This is Badger Prairie Park.

From here, the trail angles slightly to the right. When grasses are short and paths are in need of mowing, you may have to rely on trail posts. The Verona Library is visible far ahead off to the right. At 0.2 mile, the trail turns up the hill and starts heading southeast on a line to a water tower on top of the hill. Beyond here is a Dispersed Camping Area, usable only by thru-hikers.

Another 0.1 mile brings you to a playground, parking, and restrooms on your right. The trail passes the parking lot, goes under the big wooden Ice Age Trail sign, and follows a mowed path until it connects to the paved bike path. Go right and follow the trail all the way to Verona Avenue, where you will cross under via a tunnel.

On the other side, go left on the paved trail and you will come to the parking area for the Military Ridge State Trail and Ice Age Trail. There's information about the former Dane County "Poor Farm" that was once nearby. Follow along the asphalt path at the edge of the lot past a map board and picnic tables. There is a map box for this trail to your right.

LENGTH & CONFIGURATION: 6.3-mile point-to-point or 12.6-mile out-and-back

DIFFICULTY: Easy to moderate

SCENERY: Prairie, woodlands, moraines, some suburban overlooks, flowing water, ponds

EXPOSURE: Some shaded portions, a lot of sun

TRAFFIC: Light

TRAIL SURFACE: Packed dirt with tree roots, mowed paths

HIKING TIME: 2.5 hours each way

DRIVING DISTANCE: 4.2 miles southwest of Verona Road/US 18/151 and the Beltline Highway (US 12/14)

ACCESS: Year-round

MAPS: USGS *Verona; Ice Age Trail Atlas;* sometimes in map box at Military Ridge State Trail parking lot

WHEELCHAIR ACCESSIBILITY: None

FACILITIES: Restrooms and water at Reddan Soccer Fields in Verona and Badger Prairie Park; parking at trailhead, Military Ridge State Trail, and Prairie Moraine County Park

CONTACT: iceagetrail.org, 800-227-0046

COMMENTS: Be prepared for mosquitoes along Badger Mill Creek, and some of the wooded sections might call for long pants due to scratching foliage.

Continue a short way down the asphalt trail to cross a culvert, and go right on the Military Ridge State Trail. Hikers do not need to pay a trail fee, but bikers do. You'll follow the old rail bed 0.2 mile and cross a bridge before the trail goes left through grass and brush and starts south along Badger Mill Creek on the left and unrestored prairie and agricultural fields to the right. This continues for 0.4 mile, and then you'll pass a bat house on the right and enter a stand of pine. Cross the creek on a wooden bridge with metal railings as the trail goes right a short distance to another wooden bridge that crosses another smaller channel. Mosquitoes can get pretty bad through here.

The trail shows some crushed rock in a few low places; otherwise, it can get rather soupy after heavy rains from Military Ridge Trail to CR M. The next 0.5 mile gives no cover. You see a lot of grass, pine, and aspen to the right, and just brush to the left until you come to a wooden gate. To your right is a covered wooden bridge, and residences are on both sides of the trail but set back from the narrow corridor of woods and the creek, which is still on your right. Go straight across through the next gate and continue another 0.4 mile until you come to Whalen Road.

Cross Whalen Road to the opposite sidewalk, and then go slightly left and up a hill with a water tower. You'll pass a fireplug on the left near the top. Look right and over the view of condos. Facing the road, you can see Blue Mound at 1 o'clock in the distance on a clear day.

The trail continues and descends the other end of this 0.2-mile ridge. You again pass through a ditch, following trail posts along CR M. The trail uses a wide sidewalk on the overpass to get across US 18/151. At the end of the guardrail at the other side, the trail goes left to the left side of the power lines.

It runs alongside what is still CR M for just over another 0.1 mile before crossing to the right where you can see an electrical box and a trail sign. The trail leaves the roadside

Ice Age Trail: Verona Segment

Five Points

CTH PD

CTH PD

To 14

High Point Road

CTH M

Maple Grove Drive

Reddan Soccer Fields

water tower

Cross Country Road

Cross Country Road

Nesbitt Road

18 151

BADGER PRAIRIE COUNTY PARK

Military Ridge State Trail

Verona

Badger Mill Creek

Verona Avenue

Military Ridge State Trail

CTH M

Grandview Road

CTH PB

18 151

Whalen Road

Paoli Street

18 151

69

Locust Drive

Range Trail

CTH M

PRAIRIE MORAINE COUNTY PARK

dog park

Wesner Lane

CTH PB

Ice Age National Scenic Trail

N

0   0.2   0.4   0.6 mile
0   0.2 0.4 0.6 kilometer

and crosses into a low-lying field with a residence and trees to the right. Just 0.1 mile brings you to standing water on your right and a trail that bears left into the woods.

Cross a wooden bridge just inside the trees to another stagnant pond to the left. Another 0.1 mile brings you to a small land bridge through another low area, and then you pass through apple trees to agricultural fields. Go left to the corner of the field, and the trail bends right and follows along the edge of the trees. At the corner is a fence to keep you on course. From the turn, the trail crosses 0.2 mile through the field to a narrow band of oak and hickory, where it ducks in and ducks back out on the other side and goes left. It follows along another farm field. Deer can be abundant here when corn is planted.

It's only another 250 feet to the woods where the trail heads uphill moderately on a narrow footpath for another 0.2 mile before exiting the trees down a short slope to County Road PB. Go left along the road facing traffic and watch for a Do Not Enter road sign with a small yellow patch on the post. Cross to your right here and pick up the trail on the other side.

Just inside the woods, the trail goes right with scattered rocks and tree roots. CR PB is not far to the right, and a rusty fence keeps you on track from the left. This wooded stretch lasts only another 0.1 mile, and then the trail heads into the open to the left and takes a gentle curve to the right, passing under an enormous oak before heading out through oak savanna and prairie.

From the oak, it is 0.2 mile to the crest of the hill, where you will find a trail juncture marked with a white blaze. Down this path, keeping right at the next two junctures should take you up to the top of the moraine for a very nice panoramic view and a bench from which to admire it. Within here are other trails along the moraine and connections into the dog park to the south. From there, you can get out to the parking lot at Prairie Moraine County Park. If you skip the white-blazed trail at the hilltop juncture, follow the yellow-blazed trail to the right as it curves past a gate to the dog park and then switches back, descending west along the moraine until the final turn to the south before ending at a gate into the parking area at Prairie Moraine County Park, possibly the most popular dog park in the area. If you are planning on using two vehicles to make this a one-way hike, this is the place to park, where CR PB meets Wesner Lane just 1 mile south of US 18/151.

Nearby Activities

Stop in for a treat at Michael's Frozen Custard at 407 West Verona Ave. in Verona. Call 608-845-8887 or go online and see their flavor calendar at **ilovemichaels.com.** Verona's own production brewery, Wisconsin Brewing Co., is just north of Prairie Moraine County Park at 1079 American Way. They offer tours and a taproom.

GPS COORDINATES

N43° 00' 56.08" W89° 31' 13.14"

Go 1.8 miles southwest on Verona Road/US 18/151 from where it intersects with the Beltline Highway (US 12/14). Go 2.4 miles west on County Road PD to the parking area on the left. The trailhead is at the northwestern corner of the lot.

45 Magnolia Bluff Park

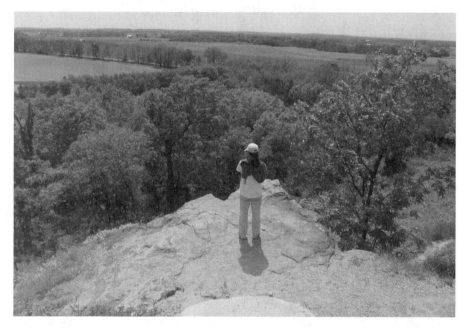

The bluff offers a magnificent view off a rock outcrop at the top.

In Brief

Trek around and to the top of an exposed rocky bluff for a fantastic view of the surrounding countryside, see some rare plants, and explore hardwood forest.

Description

Primarily consisting of sandstone, Magnolia Bluff exists as it does today thanks to a top layer of limestone that has slowed its erosion over eons. One can still see the exposed sandstone layers from the trail around the base of the bluff. But at the top is a view from the exposed rock at the western end of the hill, perfect for sunsets and a vista that extends all the way into Green County. The 120-acre park is also a designated State Natural Area, and the short grass savanna area along the western bluff top is home to the state threatened wildflower, kittentails. The park has two parking lots: The upper lot tends to draw those who are just popping by to take in the view and maybe a picnic, but the lower lot is where you'll find the trailhead.

The park trails were overhauled in 2014, so be sure to stay on the designated trails and allow the defunct paths to be absorbed back into nature. The trail starts off sandy on a moderately steep incline, crossing the southern side of the bluff on a course that

LENGTH & CONFIGURATION:
2.4-mile loop

DIFFICULTY: Moderate due to some trail surfaces and moderately steep areas

SCENERY: Mixed forest, rock outcrops, bluff-top vistas

EXPOSURE: Mostly shaded

TRAFFIC: Light

TRAIL SURFACE: Packed dirt, mowed grass

HIKING TIME: 1 hour

DRIVING DISTANCE: 6.5 miles southwest of WI 59 and Main Street in Evansville

ACCESS: 5 a.m.–10 p.m.

MAPS: USGS *Orfordville;* map posted on site

WHEELCHAIR ACCESSIBILITY: Only along the top of the bluff near the upper lot

FACILITIES: Water, pit toilets, picnic tables, and grills

CONTACT: www.co.rock.wi.us/parks-info-maps?id=465 or dnr.wi.gov/topic/Lands/naturalareas/index.asp?SNA=648

COMMENTS: Leashed dogs allowed but not in picnic areas. Hikers should yield to horses on the bridle trail portions. State Natural Area rules apply.

switches back to take you to the top near the western edge. Only 70 feet in, the sandy patches give way to a packed-dirt path through mixed hardwood forest with abundant brush. Catch glimpses of the exposed sandstone up the slope on your left. Creepers from berry bushes may reach over the trail, so beware of them and their greedy thorns. You will encounter a few short, steep moments as you come to about 0.4 mile, and the surface is a mix of dirt, sand, scattered rocks, and tree roots. You'll cross over a shallow gully descending to the right and then come upon a trail down to the right; this path takes you out to the park road as it curves to the upper lot. So go left to stay in the woods.

A couple hundred feet more and you'll see another spur trail out to the park road as the trail makes its turn back to the west. From here, it passes under that sandstone before climbing up to the bluff top. Here it heads west, with a paved trail running parallel on the right side. The two paths join and you find yourself in a shortgrass savanna with a scattering of oaks and black walnut trees. Stop to read some ecological signage there. The trail brings you right to the edge of the bluff, where the rock juts out and the elevation gives you a far-reaching view to the west. Spur trails offer a chance to step down under this rock to see it up close. This area beyond the wooden fence is home to kittentails (*Besseya bullii*), which shows small yellow flowers in a spike-shaped formation when it blooms in late May–June.

After you've enjoyed the view, follow the wooden fence along the bluff edge to where the hiking trail continues back to the east along the other side. Some large boulders have tumbled down the hill here. Trek east now on a hiking-only trail until it joins the hiking and bridle trail 0.2 mile later. (A spur trail to the right before that point heads back to the parking lot and toilets.) At the juncture with the bridle trail, a cutoff trail descends to the left, and a trail to the right leads into a gathering area for riders. Go straight across and the trail follows a gradual bend to the right until it comes to another juncture after 0.25 mile. Go left here and, in another 500 feet, pass two trails on the left;

Magnolia Bluff Park

these, too, cut across the loop, shortening the hike just a bit. Continue east, now passing through some pine, to the edge of the park where the trail turns north. (The Ice Age Trail may connect here in the future.)

Along this 0.3-mile segment, large old hardwoods lean out like archways, and colonies of aspen have gained some ground in the mix. At the north end, the trail turns west again. At this corner on the right is the park's eastern viewpoint, but when leaves are on the trees, there is nothing to see. For the next quarter mile, the trail descends on a sandy and rocky path, immediately passing the connecting trail from the south side of the loop. The understory opens up for better views inside the woods, and you will pass one trail on the right, which leads to another bridle trail loop in newly acquired park land, and two more trails on the left, the second of which zigzags back up the bluff to where you first encountered the bridle trail at the top.

Continue west from this trail juncture another 0.1 mile and you will come to another. The path to the right goes out to the northern edge of the park and follows the property line just inside the border from private fields. Better to stay left at this juncture and admire the slope of the bluff up to the left before the forest closes in a short distance later. About a half mile remains, and just before you reach the end, you come to a four-way trail juncture. From the right is that property-line path, and straight across is a short stem trail to the edge of a marshy spot alongside Croaker Road; explore, if you like. Then follow the trail to the south a short distance to the lower parking lot. A water pump stands to the right as you come off the trail.

Nearby Activities

Nearby Evansville has three historic districts listed on the National Register—three properties in particular, as well—and showcases architecture from as far back as the 1840s. Free walking-tour guides are available at city hall and several area businesses, and the Evansville Grove Society offers guided tours by appointment. Call 608-882-5528 or email grovesociety@gmail.com.

GPS COORDINATES
N42° 43' 49.61" W89° 21' 20.71"

Take US 14 south 13.6 miles from its intersection with the Beltline Highway (US 12/18) in Madison. Turn right (west) on WI 92, drive 1.5 miles, and turn left (south) on WI 104. Go 7.9 miles, turn left onto WI 59, go 0.5 mile, and then take the first right onto North Croak Road. At 0.5 mile, turn left into the parking lot and find the trailhead off the northeast corner of the lot.

46 New Glarus Woods State Park

A field of native prairie flowers

In Brief

Explore the woods south of New Glarus, which teem with wildlife. Trails run through rolling restored prairie and hardwood forest offering nice vistas, and the park's nature guide and interpretive trail make it an educational experience.

Description

The farmland around here undulates with the rolling terrain of the unglaciated corner of southwestern Wisconsin. When European settlers arrived, they interrupted the burns—natural or by American Indians—that kept the prairie and oak savanna healthy. Because of this, woods went unchecked and brush filled in beneath the tree cover. Today, some prairie sections have been restored through burns and reseeding with native species. Some of the native plant life, however, rose naturally from beneath the ashes of prescribed burns after lying dormant there for many years.

LENGTH & CONFIGURATION: 3.8-mile loop	**WHEELCHAIR ACCESSIBILITY:** Restrooms and an accessible wildlife blind on the Walnut Trail
DIFFICULTY: Moderate	
SCENERY: Prairie, mixed forest, scenic overlook	**FACILITIES:** Toilets, water, picnic tables, playground, campsites
EXPOSURE: Mostly shaded but exposed in prairie sections	**CONTACT:** dnr.wi.gov/topic/parks/ name/ngwoods, 608-527-2335
TRAFFIC: Light	**COMMENTS:** The park produces a trail guide that corresponds to numbered stations throughout the Havenridge Nature Trail. There are also shorter, easier trails, plus a paved connecting trail to the Sugar River State Trail. All vehicles require a park sticker ($7 daily, $25 annual for vehicles with WI plates). The park participates in the Junior Ranger/Wisconsin Explorer program (see Preface, page 8).
TRAIL SURFACE: Packed dirt, mowed grass, some tree roots and rocks	
HIKING TIME: 1.5 hours	
DRIVING DISTANCE: 17.5 miles from US 18/151 and WI 69 near Verona	
ACCESS: 6 a.m.–11 p.m. year-round	
MAPS: USGS *New Glarus;* brochure	

Chipmunks and ground squirrels create quite a chatter as you hike the New Glarus Woods, and you'd have to be rather unlucky not to scare up at least a deer or two. The prairie sections are vibrant with color, and savanna is beginning to come back in some places. The hardwoods attract some interesting bird species, such as the scarlet tanager and the northern oriole. The rise and fall of the trail will keep your pulse up a little, but it's nothing too exhausting.

Cross CR NN from the roadside parking lot and the trail descends with a surface of dirt and occasional tree roots. The park managers maintain the breadth of the trail with regular cutting, but the path is natural and uneven, sometimes sloping to the left or right. Numbered signposts along the route correspond to entries in the *Havenridge Trail Companion Booklet,* available free at the park office. It's informative and great for all ages, and it includes quotes from famous naturalists.

The first stretch of the trail is a long, slow descent primarily through basswoods, maples, and black walnuts. Wildflowers are abundant. At 0.2 mile, you will have come down to the edge of a fantastic prairie restoration. You can see WI 69 from here over rolling hills full of flowers in summer. The trail follows along the edge of the woods, sloping down this hill and then climbing the next into open hardwood forest another 0.2 mile farther.

The shade is short-lived; 900 feet later, you are back into the prairie following the perimeter. Coneflowers are abundant. Look left out across the prairie and see a quarry in the distance. Continue down the hill and up once more and you are back into the trees. The growth here is closer together and with smaller trunks.

When you come back into the open after 500 feet, there's a bench up ahead with an educational sign showing you the various prairie plants of southern Wisconsin, complete

with drawings. Then it's back into the woods for another 900-foot stretch. To your right is the 0.5-mile Walnut Trail, which cuts 1.1 miles off this southern loop of the Havenridge Trail and bypasses any further prairie.

The trail is open to the sky at this point. When you reach trail marker 13, 0.3 mile from the Walnut Trail trailhead, the land to your left is the beginning of oak savanna. Look carefully to see some patches of wetland where a creek runs through it.

Hike another 0.3 mile to where the trees start to thin, exposing prairie. When you finally enter the field, you are at the farthest point from the highway, and even the occasional hum of truck tires fades over the hill behind you. At 400 feet from the edge of the woods, cross a culvert that channels a small creek, almost invisible in the deep grass, and the trail starts to turn right. You can see where this water runs as a long band of trees and brush sprouts out of the middle of the prairie.

Six hundred feet later, cross the creek again and go uphill to the trees. The trail follows along their edge to the left and then passes just inside the woods with a barbed-wire fence to your left marking the end of the park property. Agricultural fields lie beyond it. This is the "quietest" part of the forest, though the chipmunks might have a different idea about that.

This section of the trail goes gradually uphill 0.8 mile to the end point of the Walnut Trail and then another 350 feet to CR NN. This is a possible cutoff point, and you could walk the highway 0.3 mile to the parking lot to your right.

Go directly across the road where the trail drops off the edge of the asphalt just like at the beginning, going downhill through forest dominated by basswood for the first 0.4 mile. Halfway down this segment, there is a cutoff trail to the right that leads to the park office, toilets, and water.

Where the trail starts to go uphill, it also begins to curve to the right. On your left will be the Vista Trail, a 0.4-mile path that descends through the woods via a few switchbacks and connects to the Bison Nature Trail, another 0.8-mile prairie loop with an enormous swing at its southern point. If you choose to extend your hike this way, you can backtrack to this point afterward or exit the Bison at its northernmost point and follow the asphalt path along the highway back up to the parking lot. That same paved trail heads back toward New Glarus to connect to the Sugar River State Trail.

Continuing past the Vista Trail, however, you come to a bench on the right and a mowed area through the brush to the left that allows you to step to the edge to view the prairie beyond. The view from this hilltop is out over the valley of New Glarus. The trail heads south again another 0.2 mile to where it follows along the ridge, with a deep gully to your left. You'll cross that gully where it comes up almost to the trail level. A cutoff trail here leads to the park office to the south (right). Go north (left) along the opposite ridge as it does a half loop around until 0.3 mile later, where you are heading south again. Here you arrive at a trail juncture. To the left, a trail leads you out to that asphalt connection to the Sugar River Trail. Stay right just a few steps more to another fork. You have a choice; either trail takes you back to the playground area near the parking lot. Along both, you will find educational signage. Because the entire loop is only 0.4 mile—you're standing at its turnaround point—you might want to do one, come back down the other, and retrace your steps out. This Basswood Nature Trail is also a nice little loop by itself, with an educational twist, if you are short on time or energy. In spring, look for jack-in-the-pulpit and wild geraniums.

Go left at this fork, and, at 0.1 mile, pass a spur trail out to a parking lot. There's a drinking fountain here, and the trailhead of that Sugar River Trail connection is to the left at the end of the lot.

You'll exit the woods 0.1 mile later near some toilets, and a playground is off to the right. CR NN is straight ahead, and you should see your car from here. The other end of the Basswood Trail is just past the playground equipment to your right.

Hikers with kids can get a Junior Explorers discovery backpack (each is themed: birds of prey, insects, etc.), available at state parks and local libraries. The packs contain guidebooks with activities for kids to work on with parents. They can turn them in to earn a free patch. Look at the park brochure for information about weekly guided nature activities.

Nearby Activities

The town of New Glarus has a strong Swiss heritage and is worth a visit. Stop by Maple Leaf Cheese and Chocolate Haus for ice cream, more than 80 locally made cheeses, and incredible homemade fudge. Call 888-624-1234 or go to **mapleleafcheeseandchocolate-haus.com** for more information. The award-winning New Glarus Brewery just across WI 69 offers self-guided tours and sampling. Check them out online at **newglarusbrewing. com** or call 608-527-5850.

GPS COORDINATES
N42° 47′ 13.18″ W89° 37′ 51.68″

From US 18/151 near Verona, go south 3.8 miles on WI 69. Go right on County Road PB for 5.1 miles; then turn right on WI 69/92 and follow it 8.4 miles through New Glarus to CR NN. Turn right and go 400 feet to find the park office. Parking is just off the county road another 400 feet past the office. The trailhead is on the left side opposite the parking area.

47 Stewart County Park

The trail enters a ravine.

In Brief

Multiple loops take you through a ravine and thick woods and over a hill of restored prairie for a fantastic view of the countryside. A spring-fed creek feeds the diminutive Stewart Lake.

Description

Stewart Park was the first park in the Dane County park system. Central to the property is Stewart Lake, which was created by a dam on a spring-fed creek. Located just north of Mount Horeb, it is nestled in at the edge of some of the residential neighborhoods but offers good wilderness and a hilltop view of the surrounding countryside.

Restrooms are located right at the parking lot. The trail begins at the end of the parking lot and follows an asphalt path from the lot right along forest. Water runs down this channel after heavy rains. There's a pavilion to the left and a playground in this mowed area.

Walk toward Stewart Lake and enter the trees at 0.1 mile, where the asphalt ends and crushed stone begins. It is mostly shaded here by the trees going up the hill to your left. Pass first some stone blocks and then some timbers holding up the earth on that side of the trail. Cattails, brush, and a few trees separate you from the lake on your left. The path

LENGTH & CONFIGURATION: 3.6 miles; 4 interconnected loops with cutoffs	the Beltline Highway (US 12/18) and Verona Road juncture
DIFFICULTY: Moderate	**ACCESS:** 5 a.m.–10 p.m.
SCENERY: Mixed forest, prairie, flowing water, lake, dam, ravine, wildflowers	**MAPS:** USGS *Cross Plains;* on a map board deep in the trail system
EXPOSURE: Half and half	**WHEELCHAIR ACCESSIBILITY:** None
	FACILITIES: Toilets, shelter, playground
TRAFFIC: Light	**CONTACT:** countyofdane.com/lwrd/ parks/stewart.aspx
TRAIL SURFACE: Packed dirt, mowed grass, short stretch of asphalt	**COMMENTS:** Dogs require a fee ($5 daily, $30 annual) and must be on a leash. Cross-country skiing also exacts a fee ($7 daily, $30 annual).
HIKING TIME: 1.5 hours	
DRIVING DISTANCE: 19.6 miles west of	

curves to the right, and you can look for some blackberries through here in August, as well as several varieties of wildflowers.

Just 0.2 mile into the woods, pass a brick pump house and see a trail sign at the head of a mowed path just beyond it. Moen Creek is to your left. The trail crosses a culvert and then bends left at a fireplug to the right of the trail.

You then come to a fork in the trail. The trail to the left is your return path. Go right through oak, hickory, and black walnut. Look for Indian pipe, a white tubelike flower that has no chlorophyll but lives off of nutrients from fungi and decaying trees. At the next fork, 0.1 mile later, go right and cross a footbridge over the creek. This is the beginning of the 0.8-mile Green Loop with a couple of steep climbs. To shorten your hike, continue straight rather than crossing the bridge.

Right after the bridge is a culvert, and then the trail goes right. The trail heads into the bottom end of a small ravine. In the ridge to your left, you can see exposed sandstone. Pass a bench on the left and come to another fork. Go left up the hill, following the direction of the ski trails. This is steep, and if you go right instead, it is just slightly more gradual in its climb to the top of the opposite ridge.

At the top, the path levels out in a small mowed area where skiers can rest after that 0.1-mile climb.

The trail curves right just inside the park and continues slightly uphill. You pass through wildflowers and the canopy opens a bit to the sky. As you come into a small piece of prairie nearly overrun by sumac, pass along the backyards of a few houses. Straight across the field is a bench. From here, the trail starts down moderately through young black walnuts and a scattering of flowers and grasses. As you come down around the curve and into another clearing, you see the terrain slope into the groove of that ravine.

At the bottom, the path curves right and then back again to cross the ravine on a land bridge. To your right, it slips down deeply. The trail bends right and follows along the

Stewart County Park

Stewart Lake

other ridge into forest again, with the land sloping to your right. You'll come to an arrow that points down and reads STEEP SLOPE, but it is actually not as steep as your ascent on the other side. You are in a wide-open space beneath the canopy, and this is a nice view of the shape of the ravine. The trail bears left at the bottom and leads you back to the bridge and the main trail.

Go right and a short trail brings you up to the main trail and continues right 0.1 mile to a four-way trail juncture where you find a map board. If you stay on your course through this clearing, taking the trail to the right, you follow the Long Yellow Loop, which is a 0.5-mile loop returning to this spot. To skip this, look for a trail to your left that goes back in the direction you came from.

The Long Yellow Loop goes uphill and crosses prairie with a nice variety of wildflowers, including coneflowers, black-eyed Susans, false sunflowers, and cup plant. It passes through a stand of pines and then brings you to some oak savanna on the right. A blue trail arrow attached to a bluebird house points the way left. Leave the woods for prairie over hilly terrain with trees to your right. The trail heads downhill to the clearing and map board to complete this loop.

Now stay right as you pass the map board, and take the trail there. It continues up through black walnuts and soon levels off into prairie 0.2 mile from the map board. The trail curves along the boundary of the park, passing a spur trail out to Blue View Drive. From there, it is another 300 feet to a cutoff trail to the left, which would take the 0.8-mile Red Loop off your hike. Going right, continue over the hill and up the next through prairie, passing a bench on your right and then a spur trail to the right to Viking Road. You reach the top of the hill just 700 feet along the Red Loop. Looking around along the horizon, it is obvious you are in the Driftless Area of Wisconsin, with its rolling unglaciated terrain. You see farms and hills in the distance and the Mount Horeb water tower to the south. Continue to the end of the field, where the trail rounds a corner to the left and heads downhill with trees and brush on either side.

At Birdhouse #12, a cutoff trail goes left along the prairie, but stay straight into the forest through tall pine. The surface is packed dirt with scatterings of hickory nuts. As the trail curves left, you lose the cover of the canopy, and as you round the bend, you meet up with the prairie alternative trail from Birdhouse #12. As you continue, the hump of the hill rises to your left, obscuring the horizon with a bulging prairie. The trail bends right along the edge of the forest and brings you to the end of the Red Loop, where there is a map board and that cutoff trail joining from the left. Go right and downhill on packed dirt at a moderate grade 0.2 mile to the beginning of the Long Yellow Loop. Look for exposed rock on the left as you descend. At the trail juncture, you see the fireplug down the trail to the right. This is the return path that leads you back out past the pump house to the parking lot.

You can walk across the dam at the north end of the lake. There is a parking lot as well as toilets. From the first parking lot, go right, continuing down CR JG. Odds are you'll see deer in the park, and, if you're lucky, you will see one of the lake's resident snapping turtles.

Nearby Activities

Stop in at the Grumpy Troll (608-437-2739) at 105 South Second St. in Mount Horeb for some craft beer, pizza, and more.

GPS COORDINATES

N43° 01' 5.65" W89° 44' 40.42"

From the Beltline Highway (US 12/18), go southwest on Verona Road/US 18/151. Drive 15.6 miles and take Exit 69 to Mount Horeb and US Business Route 18/151. Merge with County Road ID, follow it 1.4 miles to a roundabout, and take the second exit to continue on CR ID/Business Route 18/151. Continue 0.6 mile to County Road JG (North Washington Street); turn right and go 0.1 mile. Turn left on Wilson Street (still CR JG), drive one block, and then turn right onto Lake Street (also still CR JG); follow it 0.7 mile to the park entrance on the right. The trailhead is at the far end of the parking lot on the right.

48 Yellowstone Lake State Park

The Wildlife Loop along the lake

In Brief

The Wildlife Loop on a dike into the lake is brimming with activity, but the prairie and oak savanna loops over rolling hills and the paths through the woods are every bit as enjoyable.

Description

This state park offers a lot of route options. The route mapped here ties most of the trails together for one long hike. Pass the pavilion and start up the trail into the woods. This heads 0.3 mile to a trail juncture. The 1.3-mile Oak Ridge Trail lies straight ahead; the 0.8-mile Prairie Loop is to the right. There's a map board here as well as a bench.

Go straight 200 feet for the easiest of the trails. Here you find another map board and a fork in the trail. Go straight into the prairie as the trail follows along the right edge. Just 100 feet along is a spur trail to the right out to Ronnerod Lane. The trail curves left and

LENGTH & CONFIGURATION: 9.4 miles of multiple loops	**ACCESS:** 6 a.m.–11 p.m. year-round
DIFFICULTY: Easy to moderate	**MAPS:** USGS *Yellowstone Lake;* at the park office and on map boards at trail junctures
SCENERY: Wetlands, lake, mixed forest, oak savanna, prairie	**WHEELCHAIR ACCESSIBILITY:** None, but the Wildlife Loop is passable
EXPOSURE: Mostly shaded except prairie and along the dike	**FACILITIES:** Pit toilets, water, shelters, picnic areas, playgrounds, swimming area, boat launch, concessions, boat rentals
TRAFFIC: Light	
TRAIL SURFACE: Packed dirt with tree roots, mowed grass	**CONTACT:** dnr.wi.gov/topic/parks/name/yellowstone, 608-523-4427
HIKING TIME: 4 hours	**COMMENTS:** All vehicles require a park sticker ($7 daily, $25 annual for vehicles with WI plates). The park participates in the Junior Ranger/Wisconsin Explorer program (see Preface, page 8).
DRIVING DISTANCE: 45.6 miles southwest of Verona Road/US 18/51 and the Beltline Highway (US 12/14)	

then ducks into the forest on a partially shaded dirt path with lots of roots and scattered acorns. Find a clearing and a bench at the turnaround point before the trail brings you back uphill through aspen. The trail comes through a bit of oak savanna before descending on crushed rock, crossing a gully, and returning to the map board. Go right back to that first map board and then go left for the Prairie Loop.

Follow the left branch of the loop out into the sunshine. Despite the name, much of the loop actually passes through the woods rather than the prairie. The path heads to the right and follows the curve of a parking loop at the end of Ronnerod Lane until it comes around again and is heading north into some pine. The path bends right to more pine and rounds the prairie, heading down on grass into mixed forest, mostly shaded. There is some moderate uphill hiking through aspen with prairie to the right and then back into thicker woods as you return to the end of the 0.8-mile loop. Go left back down the hill to the parking lot.

Cross the road from the parking lot and go right on a grassy trail alongside the road. Pass bat houses amid tall grass and wildflowers, with the lake to the left. Pass the park office to a trail juncture and map board. This is the 1-mile Wildlife Loop. Follow this mowed path going right through aspens, mostly exposed, with brush on either side. You come to an old piece of asphalt and a trail that goes left; go straight across and down this corridor. Brush seems to block wildlife; initially, you might think "wildlife loop" was a misnomer. You come to a juncture with a snowmobile trail that goes straight or right. Go left as the trail starts to follow a dike through marsh water, dead trees, and willows, not to mention mosquitoes. You have some shade, but then you come out to open sky to follow the curving dike into the lake and back to shore 0.5 mile later. Watch for all sorts of creatures, including herons, cranes, frogs, muskrats, and many birds.

Yellowstone Lake State Park

N. Lake Road

S. Lake Road

Yellowstone River

Savanna Loop

Blue Ridge Trail

Windy Ridge Trail

D

C

E

Oak Grove Trail

Blue Ridge Trail

B

Shortcut Trail

Timber Trail

Blue Ridge Trail

A P

P

Yellowstone Lake

Prairie Loop

Ronnerod Lane

P

Visitor Center

YELLOWSTONE LAKE STATE PARK

Oak Ridge Trail

To 39 78

CRF

Lake Road

Wildlife Loop

Yellowstone River

To 151 23

0.6 mile

0.4

0.6 kilometer

0.2

0.4

0.2

0

0

When you complete the loop, go right, back to the parking area. You have the option of taking your vehicle to the next half of the trails or simply hiking 0.8 mile along the park road to the next trailhead. Yet another option is to take the Blue Ridge Trail up to the hills and the Timber Trail back down to create a meandering connection to the Oak Grove Trail. There is another parking area near the Oak Grove Trail on the left side of the road. From here, hike on the left side of the park road and continue 0.1 mile east to the trail going left into the brush. There is a map board here, and the trail goes uphill moderately 0.2 mile to the next juncture. Your return trail comes here from the right. Stay straight, passing the Shortcut Trail on the left up to Windy Ridge Trail.

Continue another 0.3 mile to the next intersection. Straight is Oak Grove and Windy Ridge Trail. Going right reduces this section of the hike to 1.3 miles on the Oak Grove Trail. Go left up the hill through moderately steep oak savanna, following a gully to the left. Find prairie as the path winds around the top end of the gully and crosses over. Another 0.2 mile takes you along the edge of the prairie and curves to a trail juncture just inside the woods. To the left is Timber Trail, which could take you back to that second parking lot to complete a 0.8-mile loop. Also a few steps in this direction is the other end of that Shortcut Trail. Go out into the prairie following Windy Ridge Trail. To your left are a parking area, a playground, and more bat houses. The trail heads 0.8 mile over the somewhat steep and rolling hills with very nice views of the land and patches of oak savanna in the distance.

The trail follows the top of a ridge, descends to the bottom, crosses the crease, and heads back up, bearing south into oak savanna. There's a bench for a rest at the top. Round some brush and savanna, remaining in open prairie until a juncture at 0.8 mile. There is a bench and a map board here. Go left on the 0.6-mile Savanna Loop. Go straight across the intersecting trail just 150 feet past here. This is the Blue Ridge Trail, where you find another map board. With farmland and barn views, the loop descends into the crease between the hills, exposed. The path goes along the left side of a small piece of savanna before curling right around it and returning up the hill, crossing back over the Blue Ridge Trail once more to the loop's starting point.

Now go left through the prairie down to more oak savanna at the bottom. Come to Point D on the park map at 0.25 mile. Go left to pick up the Oak Grove Trail. If you go right instead, it is a shorter return back down the trail you took up into the hills in the first place. Pass a short connecting spur to the Blue Ridge Trail at Point E, at 0.3 mile. This takes you to the concession stand at the southeast end of the park. The trail is mostly shaded with some open spots. As it makes its turnaround 0.6 mile later at the southernmost point of the trail, you pass a bench on the right. In the spring and fall, this is a good overlook of the lake. The next 0.4 mile offers shade and a straight moderate decline just before you cross a culvert at the bottom and arrive at the trail juncture. To the left is the path you came in on. Follow this back down to the park road and go right back to the parking lot.

The hills above the lake turn from forest to prairie.

Nearby Activities

Check out the Toy Train Barn (**whrc-wi.org/trainbarn**), a rather awesome toy train museum in a big orange barn southwest of here near Argyle. Call 608-966-1464 for current hours.

GPS COORDINATES

N42° 46' 20.86" W89° 58' 59.60"

From its intersection with the Beltline Highway (US 12/14), take Verona Road/US 18/151 southwest 19.3 miles to WI 78. Go 17.3 miles south on WI 78 through Blanchardville. On the south side of town, go right on County Road F and follow it 8.2 miles to Lake Road and the park entrance. Continue 0.8 mile south (left) on Lake Road until it brings you past the park office to the first parking area on the left. The trailhead is to the east beyond the pavilion.

NORTHEAST

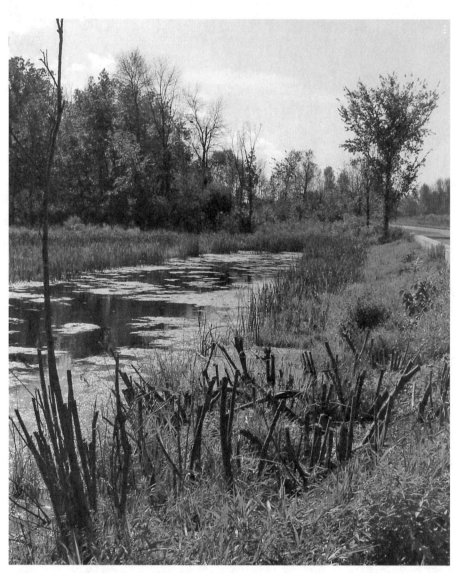

Horicon National Wildlife Refuge (see page 248)

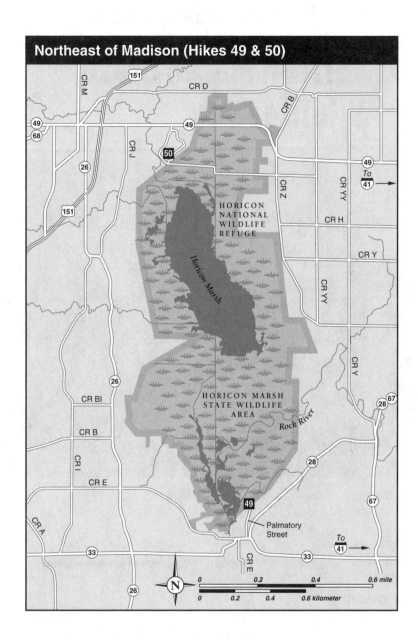

Northeast of Madison (Hikes 49 & 50)

CR M
151
CR D
CR B
49
68
49
CR J
50
26
151
CR Z
CR YY
CR H
To 41
HORICON
NATIONAL
WILDLIFE
REFUGE
CR Y
Horicon Marsh
CR YY
CR Y
26
CR BI
HORICON MARSH
STATE WILDLIFE
AREA
28 67
Rock River
CR B
CR I
28
CR E
67
CR A
49
33
Palmatory
Street
33
To 41
CR E
N
0   0.2   0.4   0.6 mile
26
0   0.2   0.4   0.6 kilometer

49 Horicon Marsh State Wildlife Area

Bachhuber Impoundment shelters abundant waterfowl.

In Brief

Walk along the dikes in one of the state's most significant bird migration points.

Description

Horicon is the largest freshwater cattail marsh in the United States; the state area alone accounts for 11,000 acres. In spring and fall, the waters teem with migrating waterfowl. To call this a quiet hike would be a lie, because geese, herons, grebes, teals, and even pelicans come in droves and create quite a bit of chatter. More than 250 species of birds pass through here each spring. Within the marsh, Fourmile Island and Cotton Island rookeries host the largest nesting colonies of blue herons and egrets in Wisconsin. There are so many birds nesting there, in fact, that the overpopulation is harming the soil and trees.

Before your hike, stop in at the Horicon Marsh Education and Visitor Center to get a birding checklist and a Junior Birder pamphlet for the kids. An abundance of exhibits on the first floor and lower level are worth seeing as well.

LENGTH & CONFIGURATION: 4.7 miles; 3 connected loops	**ACCESS:** 5 a.m.–10 p.m. year-round
DIFFICULTY: Easy	**MAPS:** USGS *Mayville South;* available in visitor center
SCENERY: Vast marshlands, waterfowl, some forest	**WHEELCHAIR ACCESSIBILITY:** Observation deck only, though the dike trail may be manageable.
EXPOSURE: Mostly sun, some shade in forests	**FACILITIES:** Two park buildings offer restrooms and water; observation decks
TRAFFIC: Light	
TRAIL SURFACE: Crushed rock, grass, and dirt	**CONTACT: dnr.wi.gov/topic/lands/wild-lifeareas/horicon,** 920-387-7860
HIKING TIME: 1.5–2 hours	**COMMENTS:** This is an **ebird.org** birding hot spot. There are special extended office hours during the migration periods. Don't forget your binoculars.
DRIVING DISTANCE: 46 miles from US 151 and I-39	

The trailhead is to the left (south) of the center when facing it from the parking lot. The trail heads out along a dike around a large portion of marsh known as Bachhuber Impoundment, which has a lot of open-water pockets sheltering hordes of waterfowl. Watch for tiny snakes and frogs on the path as well. A boardwalk runs parallel to the trail to the south, and midway across this open stretch is a cross trail to allow you to switch over to the boardwalk, if you prefer; it also connects to the island you are heading to in the next paragraph.

The dike trail curves 0.4 mile around the edge of a forested "island," leaving you at another juncture. Go left here as the trail goes onto Indermuehle Island for a 0.6-mile loop on a grassy trail through the woods. Two-thirds of the way around (if you start left), is the boardwalk trail out to the parking lot on WI 28. As you come back off the island, walk 0.4 mile west toward a pump house. At the first trail juncture, stay straight; you'll be coming back this way to follow that dike trail to your right here. At the service road, go left, and then make another quick left after that. The trail descends closer to the marsh with partial shade before you head out into the open again through prairie just a bit higher than the cattails.

First you will pass a trail on the right that cuts out to the park maintenance building and an observation deck overlooking the immensity of the marsh to the west. Stop there for the view, but then return here to the trail as it curves down around woods to the right and then runs parallel to the ridge. It ends with a turn around the end of the ridge, where it brings you to a gate at the roadside. Directly across the road is another parking lot and an alternative trailhead. Go there.

Follow cedar chips 0.15 mile through mixed forest, and emerge at the edge of the marshland. Interpretive signs lie throughout the trail. Outside the woods, a service road goes left to right; stay right as a mowed path cuts through prairie at the bottom of a sloping hill to your right. The park maintenance building and observation platform are above.

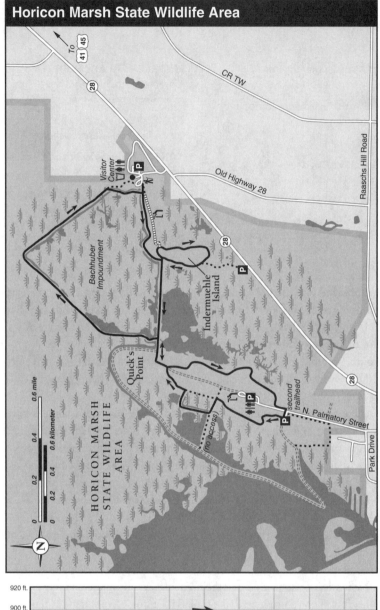

Horicon Marsh State Wildlife Area

An observation platform high on a hill affords a wide view of the marsh.

Brush will obscure the view from the trail for the first 0.15 mile, and then another 0.1 mile brings you to a trail juncture. The service road goes straight and up to the right. Go left here out into the marsh along the back of a dike. This 0.3-mile squared loop will return to the service road 0.15 mile farther north. As you venture out into the marsh, you come to a right turn at 0.1 mile; public access on the straight path beyond this point is prohibited. Marsh lies on either side of the trail. In addition to birds, be on the lookout for a lot of turtles sunning themselves.

At the end of the loop, you come back to the service road, where you go left into hardwood forest. The trail comes to a juncture at 0.15 mile. To the right is that wide service road trail again, so go left here. Another 0.1 mile takes you out of the trees and to the pump house on the left. Another much larger loop than before follows the dike north around Bachhuber Impoundment. The dike trail begins behind the pump house. The trail runs 1.5 miles out and around before returning along the bottom of the ridge behind the visitor center, where you can either take a spur trail up to the back door or return directly to the trailhead.

Nearby Activities

Dodge County Ledge Park, at N7403 Park Road in Horicon, offers overnight camping, hiking trails, and a nice overlook of the Horicon Marsh. Call 920-387-5450 to find out more.

GPS COORDINATES AND DIRECTIONS

N43° 28' 25.7" W88° 36' 4.2"

From its intersection with I-39, take US 151 north 34.3 miles to WI 33. Turn right and go 10 miles east to Horicon, staying on WI 33 as it becomes Main Street. Turn right on Lake Street, continue 0.5 mile, and then turn left on WI 28/Clason Street. Drive 1.9 miles; the entrance to the visitor center is on the left. The trailhead is just south of the center.

50 Horicon National Wildlife Refuge

The floating boardwalk on Egret Nature Trail

In Brief

Low-lying hills offer great views of prairie and wetlands, and a floating boardwalk allows access to the marsh and its bounty of wildlife.

Description

This is the federally run portion of the marsh, so there is no state park fee. It is the largest freshwater cattail marsh in the country, and birders treat this as a mecca during the migration periods, when more than 250 species pass through. In May, as many as 100 species of warblers have been recorded. The scenic park road is a 3-mile loop that can also accommodate wheelchairs. If you are looking for a short visit to the marsh, just skip to the Egret Trail and floating boardwalk right near the trailhead. Otherwise, start from the Red Fox Hiking Trail trailhead across the road from the lot entrance. There is a map posted here. Just 200 feet into the prairie, the trail forks after a short boardwalk over a low area. Go left through open prairie showing an abundance of wildflowers.

TRAFFIC: Light but moderate on the Egret Trail and boardwalk

TRAIL SURFACE: Mowed grass, crushed limestone, boardwalk

HIKING TIME: 1.5–2 hours

DRIVING DISTANCE: 52.2 miles from US 151 and I-39

ACCESS: During daylight hours year-round

MAPS: USGS *Waupun North and South;* posted in parking lots and at trailheads

WHEELCHAIR ACCESSIBILITY: Only the boardwalk and park road

FACILITIES: Pit toilets at two parking areas

CONTACT: fws.gov/refuge/horicon, 920-387-2658

COMMENTS: Dogs must be leashed and on trails. This is an **ebird.org** birding hot spot; the best times to go are during spring and fall migration seasons. A park visitor center farther east of this section of the refuge offers more information about the flora and fauna.

The trail loops 0.35 mile over the hill, passing close to some trees and then finally into the woods. The shade lasts only 0.1 mile, and then you head back into prairie. Just outside the woods, you come to the top of a hill, where there's a bench to sit and take in the view of prairie and marsh beyond.

Just down the hill another 300 feet, you come to a juncture. Going to the right returns you to the parking lot and completes the Red Fox loop. To the left is a 300-foot connection to the Redhead Hiking Trail. At this next juncture, go left through open prairie 0.2 mile to the park road. On the other side of the road, the trail continues through a row of trees before it comes into an area with cattails to the right.

The trail heads toward trees and brush, and, at 0.2 mile, you find a bench. The path bends right and downhill through open forest. At the bottom, you come to a nice little clearing that sits at the edge of some open water. There is a bench here that makes a good spot to sit and take it all in. This is a likely place to find a heron.

Another 0.1 mile leads you over another boardwalk, and then you hike along the edge of a ridge with trees to your right but no canopy. As the trail starts to climb from here, you find a bench with another good view 0.2 mile from the boardwalk. The trail passes over the top of a hill, curves right toward the forest, and then continues back down the hill to another boardwalk at 0.2 mile. Follow the path back through open prairie once more, climb another low hill, and come to a bench overlooking open water. Bring your binoculars; the birds are not that close. From the bench, it's 0.4 mile back to the park road, passing two more benches, some large cottonwoods, and a patch of trees and brush before rising up to the road.

On the other side, the trail makes a short climb and passes a boulder as you cross one more hill of prairie and 0.15 mile before arriving at the parking lot closest to the park entrance (not yours). You can find pit toilets here but, much like at the other parking lot, no water.

Go right at the edge of the lot to a service road from the corner of the lot and a small park office/kiosk, which is open only intermittently. At the corner of the lot, go left

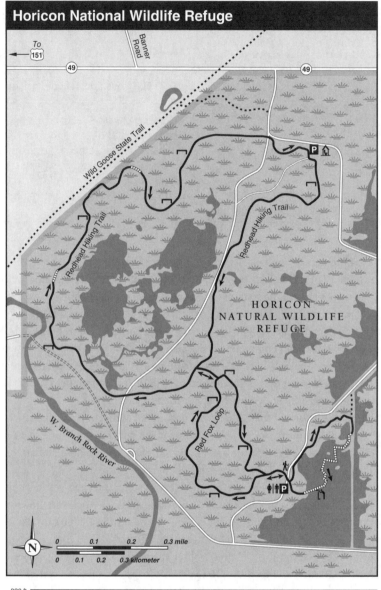

Horicon National Wildlife Refuge

HORICON
NATURAL WILDLIFE
REFUGE

midway down the side of the parking lot to find the head of the next trail segment. Continue on crushed limestone as the trail takes you through prairie 0.75 mile to the end of the Redhead Trail loop, passing close to the edge of the park road and through some brush near the end. A short pass through the woods also brings you through a gap in an old rock wall. Back when this was farmland, the farmers had to do the painstaking work of removing stones—which, thanks to the glaciers, are abundant—from the fields. From the rock wall, it's prairie until that connecting trail. Go left at the trail juncture, taking the connecting trail back to the Red Fox Hiking Trail and going left. Another 0.35 mile takes you back to the trail fork, where you go left across the boardwalk and out to the park road.

At the road, go straight across and up a short trail on a small knoll. To the right is the parking lot, and ahead are three benches. Go left on a boardwalk a few feet as it takes you at an angle to the roadside, where the crushed-rock trail and park road cross a marshy area with a low concrete curb to the right overlooking open water. There is a bench halfway across the 200-foot gap. On the other side, the trail breaks right and heads into the shade of hardwood forest. This 0.6-mile loop briefly passes through the trees and then comes out on a floating boardwalk through the cattails. Just past the trees is a trail to the left out to the road. Go right as it takes you to the boardwalk that zigzags through the marsh. Find an observation deck to the left at the first juncture. It has benches and a roof over it for shade. There is a second platform, much lower to the water and unshaded, 0.1 mile past the first one. From the end of the boardwalk, take a short asphalt path back to the parking lot.

Nearby Activities

Across the highway from the park entrance is the privately owned and volunteer-operated Marsh Haven Nature Center. There is a short trail and a 30-foot observation tower here, and the center itself offers a variety of information and houses a small museum. Admission to the museum exacts a nominal fee (about $2–$3). Call 920-324-5818 for more information.

GPS COORDINATES AND DIRECTIONS
N43° 37' 6.31" W88° 40' 15.11"

From its intersection with I-39, take US 151 north 48.1 miles to WI 49 near Waupun. Go 2.1 miles east on WI 49 to the park entrance on the right. Enter the park and drive 1.7 miles to the parking lot for the Egret Trail on the right. The trailhead is across the road from the lot entrance and marked with a sign that reads RED FOX HIKING TRAIL.

SOUTHEAST

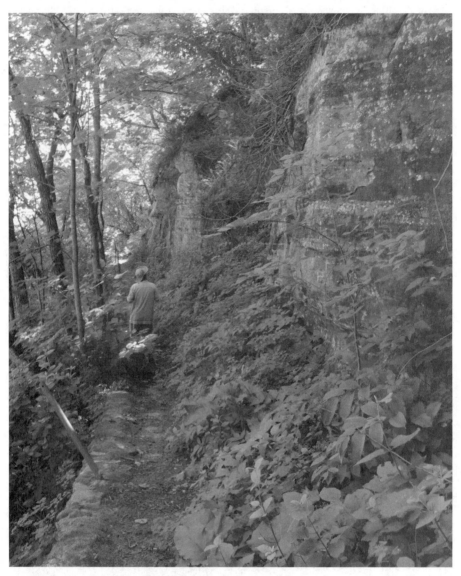

Ice Age Trail: Devil's Staircase Segment (see page 268)

Southeast of Madison (Hikes 51–60)

51 Aztalan State Park

One of the large earthen mounds, like a step pyramid

In Brief

Climb earthen pyramids at a grassy archaeological site along the Crawfish River and learn about an advanced American Indian culture that left as much mystery as artifacts.

Description

Thought you'd need to go to Egypt or Central America for pyramids? Think again. Two earthen step pyramids and the artifacts and evidence gathered here indicate this was an important site for a mysterious American Indian people.

There are remains of other temple-mound towns in the United States, but this is the farthest north of them all. Probably this tribe was related to the Cahokia, whose center was near present-day St. Louis. The Crawfish River must have been attractive to the native community as a good source of fish and wild rice, and the waterway served as a transportation route flowing south to the Rock River and farther on to the Mississippi River.

The archaeological record indicates the site was occupied between 1000 and 1300 A.D. The stockade and pyramids have been reconstructed to give an idea of the size of the community. Circular mounds can be found farther up the hill and to the north. Erroneous beliefs that this was somehow related to the Aztecs brought it the name Aztalan after it was rediscovered in 1835. The discovery of human bone fragments with animal remains

LENGTH & CONFIGURATION: 1.8-mile loop	**WHEELCHAIR ACCESSIBILITY:** Yes, but grassy trails
DIFFICULTY: Easy with a couple of short moderate climbs	**FACILITIES:** Water, restrooms, picnic tables, grills, and shelters
SCENERY: Flowing water, prairie with some mixed forest, American Indian–built earthen pyramids and mounds	**CONTACT:** dnr.wi.gov/topic/parks/ name/aztalan, 920-648-8774
EXPOSURE: Mostly exposed	**COMMENTS:** There's a designated pet area, but pets must be leashed. Visitors must pay a state park vehicle registration fee of $7 ($10 non-WI plates) or an hourly fee of $5. Educational signs throughout give valuable information about the history and archaeology of the site. A free audio guide is available online at the park website and can be downloaded as an MP3 file. Check the Friends of Aztalan site for information on free and group guided tours: **i94.biz/aztalan/aztalan.html.**
TRAFFIC: Light to medium	
TRAIL SURFACE: Mowed grass	
HIKING TIME: 1 hour	
DRIVING DISTANCE: 3.2 miles from the intersection of I-94 and WI 89	
ACCESS: 6 a.m.–10 p.m. year-round	
MAPS: USGS *Jefferson;* archaeological maps on site	

in refuse heaps has prompted some archaeologists to speculate if there was cannibalism occurring—ritualistic or otherwise—but there is no agreement on the significance of the findings. There were once more than 40 mounds here, but many of them fell under the plow before the land was turned over to the state in 1927.

After you pay your vehicle fee at the self-pay station in the parking lot at the park entrance, continue deeper into the park almost 0.5 mile to the last parking lot to find a picnic area with grills and some pit toilets nearby. Look for a water pump at the northeast corner of the lot; the trail starts here. From the pump, look east toward the river and find a posted map showing where other temple towns of mounds are located in the United States. Continuing toward the river, hike along the left side of a partial segment of stockades. (You might want to first check out the river on the right side, where the mowed grass goes right to the edge, because your opportunities will be minimal along the trail.)

The wide trail is cut grass and passes through mixed forest as it follows the river, though not directly along the shore. There's a short spur trail that leads to the water's edge just after the main trail curves left away from the stockade. Just several steps past this is an educational sign about the importance of fishing to the natives.

Within the forested section of the trail, you are sheltered from wind by thick undergrowth and woods, but there is generally no cover from the sun above. For the next 500 feet, you pass two more interpretive signs regarding hunting and gathering before reaching an opening to the field to your left. If you face the field, you can see the largest of the mounds at about 10 o'clock. Along the river to the right of the trail, swallows swoop over the muddy waters.

Seven hundred feet from here and again 200 feet past that are two more interpretive signs. Another 200 feet brings you to some shade and another section of the stockade. A

Aztalan State Park

A reconstruction of the stockade

trail goes left along the inside of it, and as you pass through a "gate" in the fortifications, you also see a trail along the opposite side. These cut back to the open field, if you just can't wait. Otherwise, continue straight along the path parallel to the river. Five hundred feet along is a short low area that can be soggy in wet weather and spring. A wood-chip cutoff trail cuts left back to the field 300 feet beyond that, and, finally, the main trail takes the turn away from the river—which has been hidden throughout most of the trail by foliage—about 0.2 mile from where you passed through the stockade.

The path becomes packed dirt and heads into more shaded territory, but the understory thins out, and you can see deeper into the trees. Just 500 feet later, you enter the clearing. A trail goes left along the trees back in the direction of the parking lot, but go straight and then keep following the trail as it bears right and follows the curve of the trees. The trail puts trees on your right and tall grass on your left; 300 feet later, it starts a moderate climb up the hillside. It's about 250 feet that brings you to the first in a row of conical mounds running south from the northwest corner of the park. Here you are at the highest point and can see the entire park and how it's laid out. Behind you are elms and locust trees, and you are a short walk from the museum. You might opt to go to the nearby county road and head north 750 feet to the museum.

Continuing from the first mound, the trail heads south alongside the uncut grass of the central field and puts the mounds to your right. You can opt to walk across the top of the mounds; it is allowed. There are 10 mounds here altogether, and they are spread out along a 500-foot stretch.

You arrive at the upper parking lot. Trails head left down the gentle slope of the land through prairie, and there's an interpretive map of the site just off the edge of the lot. Go to the end of the lot and take the trail left down the hill on a direct line to the right edge of the stockade. When you reach it, follow left along the outside of the tall wooden poles until the corner, and then continue along the stockade to the bottom of the hill. There are spaces between the poles, and you can cut through here and approach the mound within the walls from below, rather than just come around the stockade at the very beginning. It makes more of an impression this way. If you don't cut through the stockade, you can continue into the woods to where you originally passed through the wide "gate" as you walked the forest trail, and then come back up on the other side.

Once inside the stockade, turn back up the hill. Tucked into the corner is a large squared mound with steps up the center of it. Follow the trail up the hill and climb to the top of the mound. Return to the trail either by the steps or just by hiking down the steep backside. Now you can continue south off the end of the stockade, crossing the field along a series of interpretive signs until you arrive at the largest of the mounds, a sort of earthen step pyramid also shielded by reconstructed stockade. Trails crisscross the open field within the reconstructed and imagined stockades, but they will change according to park mowing patterns. Out here in the open, however, the landmarks of earth mounds and stockades and even interpretive signs are easy to spot. The distance from the first pyramid to the far side pyramid is 0.2 mile.

This second construction is the larger of the two. Originally, the top was shielded from view for sacred ceremonies. Pass behind the mound to find an interpretive sign and then go around to the front to steps going up each of the two pyramid levels. The view from the top is another nice impression of the entire site and a good photo opportunity.

From the base of the front of the mound, cross the open field to a low hill where there is an interpretive shelter/kiosk. You will learn much more about the history and excavation of the site here. From here, follow one of the mowed paths 600 feet back to the parking lot.

Guided tours are given on weekends April–October. Schedules are posted at the park, or call the park office in Lake Mills at 920-648-8774. This National Historic Landmark shouldn't be missed.

Nearby Activities

The Aztalan Historical Museum is right next door and includes some area artifacts, as well as a collection of antiques. It is open mid-May–September, Thursday–Sunday, 1–4 p.m. You can contact the museum at 920-648-4362.

GPS COORDINATES AND DIRECTIONS

N43° 03' 48.33" W88° 51' 42.64"

Exit I-94 at WI 89 (Exit 259) and go south. Turn left at the traffic light on County Road V and go 2 miles to CR B. Go left here 0.7 mile and turn right on CR Q. The museum is on your left, and the park entrance is another 0.3 mile ahead on the left. Follow the park road to the last parking lot to find the trailhead.

52 CamRock Park: Area 2

Koshkonong Creek meanders through wetland.

In Brief

A pleasant path through pine and oak forest also takes you on a loop of marvelous prairie restoration and then along the Koshkonong Creek, where it meanders through the wetlands of what was once the Rockdale Millpond.

Description

Many of the hikes in this book expose you to prairie restorations, but this park features a restoration of a different sort. Removal of the Rockdale Dam, which had once held back a large mill pond that flooded much of the area behind the present-day park, allowed the Koshkonong Creek to find its narrow way again. In almost no time at all, the resulting mud flats were once again thriving with plant life and abundant wildlife. The removal of the dam has also improved fish migration. One hundred dams have been taken out of Wisconsin waterways since 1967, and in many cases this has meant the restoration of valuable ecosystems.

There are actually three separate parks under the name of CamRock, so be sure you have gone to Area 2. You can view the path on a map board at the trailhead. Enter the

LENGTH & CONFIGURATION: 2.2-mile loop with an embedded loop	**ACCESS:** 5 a.m.–10 p.m.
DIFFICULTY: Easy	**MAPS:** USGS *Rockdale;* at trailhead on a map board
SCENERY: Mixed forest, prairie, wetlands, flowing water	**WHEELCHAIR ACCESSIBILITY:** None
EXPOSURE: Mixed	**FACILITIES:** Shelter, restrooms, water, playground
TRAFFIC: Light	**CONTACT:** countyofdane.com/lwrd/parks
TRAIL SURFACE: Packed dirt, mowed grass	
HIKING TIME: 1 hour	**COMMENTS:** Leashed dogs allowed but with a fee. Biking and cross-country ski-ing exact trail fees as well. There are three separate sections of park along County Road B, and all of them have trails.
DRIVING DISTANCE: 16.3 miles east of I-39/90/94 and US 12	

woods under a sign across the trail; at the first fork, go left, following the arrow on a trail sign. The trail follows the direction of the park road deeper into the park, and within just 400 feet, you pass under a large oak and enter open prairie with a vast number of restored prairie flowers. Initially, the view is blocked by brush and the park road is visible close by on the left. Pass a stand of aspens on your right and a mammoth oak to the left, and then the trail becomes grassy as it heads uphill. The field explodes with bergamot, coneflow-ers, Queen Anne's lace, and black-eyed Susans in the summer months. Crest a small hill and find a couple of benches next to a small oak. This is a good vantage point to view the colorful field before you.

Head down the hill on the other side with the prairie to the right. At the next trail intersection, go right as the trail loops 0.2 mile through the prairie and back to this spot. You may find some posted poetry on the trail written by local schoolchildren and inspired by the natural beauty of the park. On the other side of the field, you come to a trail inter-section. Go left. This is actually the return trail going right, but take only a few steps until the return of the prairie loop cuts back into the grass and flowers and follows along the edge of the trees. When you come back to the origin of the prairie loop, go right. (The straight path is a stem out to the park road.)

You'll see another trail to the right, 200 feet later, leading to a clearing around a fire pit. This is also a cutoff trail through to your return trail. To the left is the parking area in the small park-road loop. Just past this trail is a park maintenance road that goes right and also could be a cutoff to the return. A metal gate blocks entry from unauthorized vehicles.

The main trail continues uphill and enters some Norway pine up to the top of the hill. A spur trail goes left to the shelter house, where you can find restrooms and water. There's also a horseshoe pit and playground in that open mowed area.

Staying on the main trail, pass another cutoff to the right and stay left on a trail car-peted with rust-colored pine needles. Taking the cutoff would shave 0.3 mile off your

A butterfly in bergamot

hike. When you reach an opening to the mowed area, you see a trail marker that points to the right. Follow it; the opening to the left leads out to that playground.

Pine gives way to maple as the trail curves around just inside the park boundary at the county road. There are spur trails out of the park to the left. The path descends easily and at the bottom curves right and switches back. Through the brush to your right, you can see the return trail at a lower level before you reach the curve.

On the return path, look out through the trees to your left to see cattails where once there was a mill pond. Find a bench on the right to enjoy a bit of oak savanna and wetlands beyond, while you can still breathe in the scent of pine trees at your back.

There's a bench at the opposite end of the cutoff trail. Continue past that trail and descend from savanna to the edge of the wetlands. Wildflowers find root here in the shade of the oaks. The path goes down moderately and enters aspens 200 feet later. The canopy thins here as you come around the bend, but then the trail curls right and heads north into thicker cover. A bench on the right 0.3 mile from the cutoff looks out over cattails and wet prairie. You can see across to the pavilion of CamRock Area 3.

Eight hundred feet beyond this is a mowed area through the brush to the left, where you can see out over the muddy banks of the creek. Koshkonong Creek has a bit of current to it, kicking up muddy waters. You can go right to the edge.

At the next trail juncture, you can see straight to the gate at the parking lot. Go straight to stay on the trail. To the left is a path that crosses the river on a bridge and connects this trail system to the multiuse CamRock Trail, which runs 2.4 miles from Cambridge to Rockdale. But stay here in Area 2, and the path follows along the edge of terra firma, while soggier land is just to the left of the narrow line of trees. Pass the cutoff trail on your right that leads back to the fire pit.

You enter prairie once again 0.2 mile from the opening to the creek. Go straight across, with the trees and brush to your left, passing the two segments of the prairie loop to your right. Once on the other side of the prairie, the trail goes closer to the edge of the wetlands again, and the brush thins to reveal the marsh beyond. There's a bench facing the marsh, and you can sit with the prairie right up behind you, arguably the better view.

From here, the trail is 15–20 feet above the level of the wetlands. It enters the woods again, curves right, switches back, and brings you to an observation platform 400 feet down the trail on your left and now at about marsh level. Spend some time here looking for marshland wildlife. The trail turns back toward the county road and follows along the edge of a finger of marsh to your left for another 800 feet. Canadian hawkweed is abundant along here.

The trail turns into the woods once more and follows just shy of the roadway until it brings you back to the first fork you passed near the entry. Go left here to arrive back at the parking lot.

The other two sections of the park offer more trails, although Area 3's paths are aimed more toward mountain bikers.

Nearby Activities

Cambridge is a popular tourist draw with its Victorian storefronts and a surprising collection of shops and galleries. The public beach at Lake Ripley is a good place for a swim after your hike. The town hosts Cambridge Pottery Festival and U.S. Pottery Games (**cambridgepotteryfestival.org**) the second full weekend in June of each year.

GPS COORDINATES AND DIRECTIONS
N42° 58' 41.33" W89° 01' 22.57"

From I-39/90/94, follow US 12 for 14.4 miles east to Cambridge. Halfway through town, turn right on CR B and drive 1.9 miles south to the park entrance on the right (west) side. Park in the first parking area on the left side near the entrance. The trailhead is behind you.

53 Glacial Drumlin State Trail

The bridge over Rock River

In Brief

Cross the Crawfish and Rock Rivers and get a close look at a glacial drumlin on this converted rail bed that offers a mostly shaded path through rich farmland.

Description

A glacial drumlin is a hill of debris left by a retreating ice mass. The hill rises up sharply at the front and then tapers off at an easier slope in the direction of the glacier's retreat. You see some on this hike. Glacial drumlins contain rock and gravel all the way from Canada, and, because of this, they are popular sources for the crushed rock. Quarrying has caused many drumlins to disappear.

LENGTH & CONFIGURATION: 13.2-mile out-and-back	**ACCESS:** Year-round anytime
DIFFICULTY: Easy	**MAPS:** USGS *Lake Mills* and *Jefferson*; at the trail office; **glacialdrumlin.com**
SCENERY: Farmland, wildflowers, two rivers, glacial drumlins	**WHEELCHAIR ACCESSIBILITY:** Yes
EXPOSURE: Mostly shaded with some exposed stretches	**FACILITIES:** None on trail. Restrooms and water at the trailhead.
TRAFFIC: Moderate	**CONTACT:** glacialdrumlin.com, 920-648-8744
TRAIL SURFACE: Crushed limestone	**COMMENTS:** Dogs must be on a leash no longer than 8 feet. A state trail pass is required for bicyclists age 16 and older ($4 daily, $20 annual), but no hiking fee. Stay alert for approaching bicyclists or, when snow is present, snowmobiles.
HIKING TIME: Up to 5 hours	
DRIVING DISTANCE: 21.1 miles east from the interchange of I-39 and I-94	

The entire Glacial Drumlin State Trail runs 52 miles, from Cottage Grove all the way east to Waukesha. In 1986, it was developed from an unused section of railway, so the grade is gentle. The section mapped out here is arguably the best part of the trail. It begins at an old railroad depot in Lake Mills, where you can find a small exhibit of local history, and crosses two rivers before it ends where the trail goes on road just before the city of Jefferson.

To hike both rivers and avoid the long out-and-back, you can either use two cars, parking one at the other trailhead near Jefferson, or hike from the Jefferson end of the trail. The out-and-back distance to see both river crossings is 6.7 miles from that end.

The trail begins from the depot heading east across County Road A/Main Street. After 0.1 mile, you enter shade as the rail bed sinks into the surrounding terrain. A short distance later, the surrounding terrain is lower and the trail then rides above it.

At 1 mile from the trailhead, you come out into the open for 0.3 mile before the trail finds shade again. At that point, there is a snowmobile trail heading left. Stay straight. Though there are cornfields on either side, the trail itself enjoys a corridor of mixed forest throughout much of this hike, so exposure is less than you might expect.

You pass a stand of aspens and some big cottonwoods that border the fields to the north and then a yield sign for a farm road crossing the trail. Pass through box elders to Harvey Road. The trail continues on the other side, and, 0.2 mile later, you come to an interpretive sign about glacial drumlins. You can see one to the south. The trail is exposed from here, passing through fields of goldenrod 0.2 mile to the next crossing at Mansfield Road. Beyond this road, the trail goes under the canopy of black walnuts and crosses a farm road at 0.2 mile. To your right just past here, look for a drumlin covered in prairie flowers.

Cross CR Q. To the north 1.5 miles is Aztalan State Park, an archaeological site and another nice hike. There is no official public parking on this road. On the other side, pass

Glacial Drumlin State Trail

a small bit of wetlands on the left and, soon after that, another farmer's crossing. You will go 0.3 mile from CR Q before coming to the first bridge. This is an old railroad trestle modified with wood planks to make a trail crossing 40 feet above the Crawfish River. An interpretive sign at the center of the bridge puts time and history in perspective. You can see woods on either side of the river and hear birds, crickets, frogs, the whispering wind, and even jumping fish. It's a nice place to linger a bit.

The next 0.5 mile takes you to Popp Road, with open sky and a lot of wildflowers along the way. On the other side of the road, the trail heads back into forest and grows thicker, making this one of the better places to spot woodland creatures. It's another 1.7 miles to the next road crossing, mostly shaded with a few colonies of aspen along the way. Cross CR M and enter woods again, continuing 0.2 mile to the next bridge. This is the Rock River, which eventually receives the Crawfish River downstream and continues through Illinois all the way to the Mississippi River. It was an important riverway for American Indians, connecting communities from Wisconsin to many others far downstream in the Midwest. The trail uses another former railroad trestle to make the crossing.

Past the bridge 800 feet, you pass a gravel access road to the right, and then the trail goes under the WI 26 overpass. It turns right and follows along between the highway and agricultural fields 0.3 mile to the end of the trail. There is parking here and a map board. The overpass is a good turnaround point if you are hiking back to Lake Mills. The trail does continue from the parking lot, but this is an on-road portion heading east. This last stretch is noisy being next to the highway, but it's not a bad alternative starting point for the hike.

Nearby Activities

The Zeloski Marsh Unit of the Lake Mills Wildlife Area is recently restored wetlands and an excellent bird-watching site. Sandhill Station State Campground has 15 walk-in tent sites in a secluded oak savanna 1 mile south of Lake Mills on Mud Lake Road. Call 920-648-8774 for more information or to make a reservation.

GPS COORDINATES AND DIRECTIONS
N43° 32' 34.82" W87° 50' 11.45"

From the interchange of I-39/94, go east 19.1 miles to the WI 89 exit and go right (south) 2 miles to the Glacial Drumlin State Trail Office. The trailhead is across the highway on the left.

54 Ice Age Trail: Devil's Staircase Segment

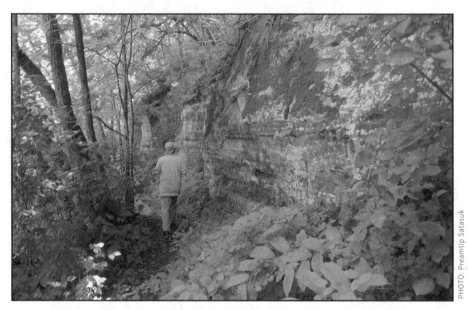

PHOTO: Preamtip Satasuk

The Ice Age Trail passes along a narrow path on the side of a bluff over the Rock River near Devil's Staircase.

In Brief

This hike combines two Ice Age Trail segments. It first passes through an arboretum along a country creek and then winds along the Rock River below sandstone cliffs and a collection of rocks resembling a giant staircase.

Description

The namesake of this hike is a geological formation that lies at the heart of the route, a collection of large stones and rock shelves resembling stairs down a ridge into the Rock River. But this hike actually combines two distinct but connected segments of the Ice Age National Scenic Trail: the Arbor Ridge and Devil's Staircase Segments. With parking at either end, it works well with two vehicles or a bike ride back to the car, but its beauty makes it worth an out-and-back trek. The 160-acre Robert O. Cook Memorial Arboretum, a popular birding destination, is the starting point at the west end, while a railway corridor easement connects the trail to the ridge along the Rock River as it enters Riverside Park at the eastern end. The Ice Age Trail then continues through the city of Janesville from there.

LENGTH & CONFIGURATION: 2.8-mile point-to-point or 5.6-mile out-and-back	**DRIVING DISTANCE:** 35 miles from the intersection of US 12/18 and I-39/90
DIFFICULTY: Moderate to difficult, with some steep portions and a narrow footpath on a steep, rocky slope	**ACCESS:** 5 a.m.–11 p.m.
	MAPS: USGS *Janesville West; Ice Age Trail Atlas;* map boards on site
SCENERY: Flowing water, mixed forest, some prairie, rock outcrops	**WHEELCHAIR ACCESSIBILITY:** None
EXPOSURE: Mostly shaded	**FACILITIES:** Water, restrooms, picnic tables, grills, and shelters
TRAFFIC: Light	**CONTACT: iceagetrail.org,** 800-227-0046
TRAIL SURFACE: Packed dirt, gravel, stone	**COMMENTS:** Dogs not allowed in the Riverside Park or Cook Arboretum portions May 15–October 15. Must be leashed otherwise.
HIKING TIME: 2.5 hours	

From the trailhead at a wooden arch that reads Jolyn Beeman Memorial Trail, walk along a paved path heading east. On the left, you will pass an alternative doubletrack path of crushed rock that, like the IAT, heads north through the arboretum. This trail would take you past the park's learning center and toilets on a wide path downhill. But continue on the asphalt and you will pass a pioneer cabin from the mid-19th century on your left. The city purchased it from an Amish family and reconstructed it here in 2000. Across the path from it is a mowed area backed by prairie flowers to the south. Continue down the path to find the Ice Age Trail where it heads into the forest on a narrow packed-dirt footpath on the left. Posts with the mammoth emblem of the trail organization, as well as yellow blazes on trees and posts, clearly mark the trail along its length.

After 75 feet, the park's nature trail joins from the left and you continue along a curve to the right through mixed forest. It comes back around and 800 feet later passes another trail juncture on the left, a return route for that nature trail. Continue past this and soon on the left you will see short spur trails into the central activity center, where classes, groups, and events are scheduled for ecological experiences. Continue past, and the trail takes a hard turn to the right and continues descending in short but moderately steep slopes. At 0.9 mile into the hike, the trail levels off and joins that previous doubletrack path coming down the hill from the left. At the 1-mile mark, the trail starts to run alongside Marsh Creek, which flows in from the west. A footbridge crosses the water to the left to a very small network of unofficial paths on the opposite bank. Explore a bit or just continue on the Ice Age Trail as it takes a slow turn to the east, with the creek never far off to the left.

After another 0.1 mile, pass a short alternative loop path on the left, which stays closer to the creek and rejoins the main trail just a couple hundred feet later. At 1.3 miles, the trail enters a meadow area and passes under power lines. A footpath follows these straight south out to Arbor Ridge Way, just a short walk from the end of that first asphalt path, if you want to cut this short.

Ice Age Trail: Devil's Staircase Segment

From here, the trail leaves the arboretum and follows midway up a slope along a forested ridge; after 0.6 mile, it comes out onto Northridge Drive. Go left here and watch for yellow blazes on streetlights. Just before the next street, the trail cuts through the prairie section there and then crosses Washington Street, where you can see a train viaduct to the left. You've already gone about 2.1 miles. On the other side of the street is the trailhead for the Devil's Staircase Segment, with parking and a map board. Starting this hike here would shorten the one-way distance to 1.7 miles.

Cross the lot and follow the trail as it passes through a small stretch of woods and brush until it arrives at the edge of Riverside Golf Course. Be careful not to distract golfers, and as you pass behind one of the greens, be aware of any incoming shots. The trail crosses the tracks to the left and then follows the fence line to the right on an asphalt path. A sign directs you under power lines to the left, and the trail slips into the brush behind one of the holes. Pass a stone bench and follow a narrow dirt path down a steep slope overlooking the Rock River. Descend a short series of steps—normal ones, not the Devil's—and you will come down closer to water level, where there is a staircase gully, crossing from right to left to the river. The large rocks here appear as steps, giving rise to the feature's name. There is rarely water here.

Cross the staircase gully and a sandy path takes you around a turn where a couple of benches await. From here, follow uneven, natural sandstone steps, which can be tricky with the loose sand on them. While the "staircase" is the headliner, the exposed sandstone along this stretch really steals the show. The path is quite narrow and the steep slope to your left may make some hikers nervous. At the narrowest and steepest spots, a thick wire strung along metal poles planted in concrete anchors provides a potential handhold. To the right is the bare rock, at some points rising up like a cliff more than 40 feet above. The trail slowly gains elevation and then follows the ridge to a long staircase down into Riverside Park. From the Devil's Staircase to these steps is about 0.5 mile. A spur trail continues into the forest above the stairs but goes only to the edge of the golf course. The Ice Age Trail continues from the bottom of the steps, following the Rock River on various trails through Janesville. This is the turnaround point for the hike as written, and restrooms and water are available near the stairs.

Nearby Activities

For some really marvelous flowers and plants, pay a visit to the 20-acre Rotary Botanical Gardens (1455 Palmer Drive, 608-752-3885, **rotarybotanicalgardens.org**).

GPS COORDINATES AND DIRECTIONS
N42° 42' 24.31" W89° 4' 17.17"

From its intersection with US 12/18, take I-39/90 south 28.9 miles to Janesville and take Exit 171A for WI 26. Merge onto Milton Avenue, continue 2.3 miles, and turn right on Memorial Drive. At 1.2 miles, turn left onto County Road A. Go 1.9 miles and turn right on Bluebird Trail. Follow it to the first parking lot on the right, and the trailhead is there.

55 Ice Age Trail: Whitewater Lake Segment

At the turnaround point of the hike lies Whitewater Lake.

In Brief

Another excellent segment of the national scenic trail, this path climbs moraines through Kettle Moraine State Forest's Southern Unit before ending at Whitewater Lake.

Description

This segment of the Ice Age Trail (IAT) heads south from US 12, but another portion heads north from the parking lot as well. Cross the highway with care, because traffic comes quickly through here. From the end of Sherwood Forest Road, go directly across to the trail marker and a metal gate across the entrance. Just after it, the trail forks. To the left is the Moraine Ridge Trail, a state horse and snowmobile trail. The narrow footpath to the right is the Ice Age Trail. It climbs a ridge through brush and on broken rock and packed dirt, moving parallel to the highway and offering good elevation in only about 400 feet.

The path then turns south, quickly leaving traffic behind. Find wood-beam and earth steps to an aspen colony, and then enter a clearing with a bench overlooking the surrounding area from the top of the ridge. Head back into the woods 100 feet later via steps down through more aspen. Brush thins out and, 0.25 mile from the bench and overlook, oaks start to dominate. The path follows along the top of moraines with good shade and nice views into the creases between them. Wildflowers appear along the trail from spring to fall. The path has a lot of stray rocks, which can make footing tricky when the leaves fall and cover them. The first moraine is about 0.2 mile long. When you arrive at the end of it, follow the trail down and then up again along the back of another lower and shorter

LENGTH & CONFIGURATION: 8.9-mile out-and-back	**ACCESS:** 6 a.m.–11 p.m. unless you are a registered camper
DIFFICULTY: Moderate to difficult	**MAPS:** USGS *Whitewater; Ice Age Trail Atlas*
SCENERY: Moraines, mixed forest, Whitewater Creek and Lake	**WHEELCHAIR ACCESSIBILITY:** None
EXPOSURE: Mostly shaded	**FACILITIES:** Portable toilet at trailhead; toilets, water, telephone, campsites at Whitewater Lake Campground
TRAFFIC: Light	
TRAIL SURFACE: Packed dirt with abundant rock and tree roots	**CONTACT:** iceagetrail.org, 800-227-0046
HIKING TIME: 4 hours	**COMMENTS:** Leashed dogs allowed. All vehicles require a park sticker ($7 daily, $25 annual for vehicles with WI plates) to park in either Whitewater Lake Campground or the Ice Age Trail lot on US 12.
DRIVING DISTANCE: 45.2 miles from the juncture of I-39/90 and US 12/18	

moraine. Another 100 feet brings you to the next one. As the moraines shrink, continue downhill until you come to the edge of a clearing 1.1 miles from the trailhead.

The trail then starts left up the hill along the clearing where high-tension lines come over the hills. The trail passes partly through the brush and hardwood forest along the edge of the clearing before cutting right across under the lines and back into forest on the other side. Cross to the other side of the hill, and then walk along the edge of a ridge heading east until the path heads right, away from the hill and into pine forest. The path is carpeted with needles, easy, and level. Come to an access road that heads to the right (south) along the edge of these tall pines. Follow it 0.1 mile to another intersection where the taller pines end on your right. Continue straight and pass through shorter pines as you follow the road to where it bends right and takes you out to Esterly Road, 0.2 mile from the last juncture. The IAT joins the horse and snowmobile trail through here. Cross the road and continue to follow the yellow trail patches. Pass through a clearing amid a lot of brush, and then take steps down through a corridor of pine.

At 0.4 mile from Esterly Road, the pines give way to oaks and aspen on the left. You can look down the ridge on both sides. Another 0.3 mile brings you to another crossing of the Moraine Ridge Trail. Take a soft right down a path marked with a sign that reads HORSES AND SNOWMOBILES PROHIBITED IN THIS AREA. Pass sumac to your left under an open sky, and continue downhill 0.1 mile on rocks and more wood beam–and-earth steps before the path switches back to lead you to CR P. Go straight across to pick up the trail, which heads into another clearing full of sumac followed closely by pine forest. Just 0.15 mile from CR P, the trail starts uphill on wood-beam steps through mixed hardwoods to pine at the top of the bluff. This segment of the trail again climbs moraines, and the path shows a lot of roots and rocks and some occasional wood-beam steps, but also offers good shade.

It's a total of 0.9 mile from the road to where you come off the back of the ridge to a scenic overlook. There is a bench here with a view of Whitewater Lake, where you'll end

Ice Age Trail: Whitewater Lake Segment

up. Steps to the right lead down the slope 300 feet to a spur trail that enters the camp-grounds. Continue past, passing the edges of the campsites just up to the right. From the spur trail, you have 0.3 mile to hike until you come to Hi Lo Road. Pass a trail to the park office, a map box, likely unstocked, and a couple of small kettles to the right and left before you come to the road crossing. To the left 200 feet is Kettle Moraine Drive. Go straight across Hi Lo Road and up into pine forest to a trail juncture 150 feet into the trees. The straight path is your return; go right into oak and pine. The trail is easier through here and mostly shaded. At 0.3 mile, cross the horse path once more, and then 0.1 mile takes you out of the forest at Whitewater Creek, which meanders through wet prairie. There is a bench here. Go right along the edge of the forest to reach a boardwalk and bridge over the small stream. On the other side is another bench. The trail goes left and bends right into the trees, crossing 200 feet to Clover Valley Road. There is an area map on the back of the road sign. Your choice now is to either turn around and head back the way you came or continue to the lake to make a small end-loop before hiking back on the IAT.

Go left 0.25 mile on the shoulder of the road to the edge of the lake on Kettle Moraine Drive. Go left again toward Whitewater Lake Recreation Area. Be careful: There's not much of a shoulder on the road here. Be sure to walk facing traffic. The lake drains under the road into Whitewater Creek, a stream with waters favorable for trout. Just past the creek, the horse trail heads left into the woods. Then 0.2 mile from Clover Valley Road, find a blue-marked trail left into the pine forest. Two hundred feet into the trees, find the IAT once again. Go right and retrace your steps to the trailhead. Alternatively, you could park a second vehicle here at the campgrounds or even stay the night if you packed equipment. The campground has pit toilets but no showers.

Nearby Activities

Rice Lake Nature Trail is a half-mile loop around an isolated section of the northeast corner of the lake. You can walk here from where the IAT crosses Hi Lo Road. Go south to Kettle Moraine Scenic Drive, then go left (east) to State Park Road and follow south to the trail's parking lot on the right at State Park Drive. Old World Wisconsin (S103 W37890 WI 67, Eagle; **wisconsinhistory.org/oww;** 262-594-6301) is a 600-acre outdoor museum dedicated to Wisconsin rural history. Various farmsteads represent several of the cultures that settled near here, and trams connect them. It is open May 1–October 31.

GPS COORDINATES AND DIRECTIONS
N42° 48' 14.26" W88° 39' 9.38"

From its intersection with US 12/18, go south 20.8 miles on I-39/90 to Exit 163 for Milton/Edgerton. Take WI 59 east (right at the end of the ramp) 2.8 miles to County Road N for 10.8 miles where it becomes Walworth Avenue outside Whitewater. Turn right on US 12 and follow it 6.5 miles to the intersection of Sherwood Forest Road. The Ice Age Trail parking lot is on the left. The trailhead is on the south side of the highway, opposite the lot.

56 Kettle Moraine State Forest: John Muir Trail

In Brief

A challenging trail climbs up and down through oak and pine forests along the rubble deposits of the last glaciers.

Description

Don't let the mountain bikers discourage you: This is a hiking trail as well. The abundance of ridges and kettles offers challenges to boots and wheels alike, and the extensive trail system leaves plenty of room for everyone. Watch for deer and turkey, as well as many songbirds.

Walking into the trail system from the trailhead, take the first right. You must go against bike traffic for safety. This trail cuts 0.1 mile to the actual loop in the same way that the leftbound trail does in the opposite direction. Between the two trails is 0.1 mile of the trail. At the juncture, go right to stay in the proper trail direction, heading north.

At 0.15 mile, the Red Trail comes from the left. You could cut 1.5 miles off the hike by going west here, taking a right 0.4 mile later on the Orange Trail, and following that up and across to connect back to the Blue Trail. This is one route (but not the only one) that can get you to the Pioneer Lime Kiln, believed to be from an 1843 Norwegian settlement called Skoponong.

Continuing on the Blue Trail, you may find the next 0.4 mile rather tame but then getting rockier and more rugged as the path climbs up a ridge. Pass a wooden fence on the right 0.5 mile from the Red Trail juncture. From there, it's another 1 mile, following a few switchbacks along the mostly shaded narrow ridge, until it comes to the connecting trail to the Emma Carlin trail 5.75 miles away. There's a map board here; stay left on the Blue Trail.

The trail switches back south, and you pass another wooden fence at 0.15 mile as you enter red pine forest for the next 0.3 mile. On the other side, you come to a fire lane crossing. There's a map board here. The Blue Trail goes straight across. You could turn left and go 0.25 mile to get to the Orange Trail and then east to the Pioneer Lime Kiln. Another 0.4 mile on the Blue Trail takes you past a glacial bog on the right and on to the Orange Trail as well, where you can go left (east) toward the lime kiln. There's a map board there.

The next juncture is 1.1 miles away. Along the path, you cross intermittent prairie patches, and then as you head into the woods, you come upon open water on either side of the trail. These are also glacial bogs. The kettles formed when ice trapped in glacial deposits melted. These particular kettles have filled with water and formed leatherleaf bogs. Just past them, the trail starts to climb and become more rugged. The path follows along a ridge with rocks along the trail edge overlooking a deep hollow to the right. Finally, you arrive at the trail juncture. To the left, the Green Trail continues and acts as a

LENGTH & CONFIGURATION: 9.5-mile loop	**MAPS:** USGS *Little Prairie;* at park office; posted at trail junctures
DIFFICULTY: Moderate to difficult	**WHEELCHAIR ACCESSIBILITY:** None
SCENERY: Mixed forest, some prairie, glacial landscape	**FACILITIES:** Pit toilets, water, picnic shelters and grills, vending machine, pay phone
EXPOSURE: Mostly shaded with some stretches of sun	**CONTACT: dnr.wi.gov/topic/parks/ name/kms/trails.html,** 262-594-6200
TRAFFIC: Light to moderate	**COMMENTS:** This trail is popular with mountain bikers, especially on weekends. Bikers must ride in one direction; be sure to go the opposite way. All vehicles require a park sticker ($7 daily, $25 annual for vehicles with WI plates). Hiking is free, but bikers must purchase a state trail pass ($4 daily, $20 annual).
TRAIL SURFACE: Packed dirt, abundant rocks and tree roots, some sand	
HIKING TIME: 4 hours	
DRIVING DISTANCE: 45.2 miles from the juncture of I-39/90 and US 12/18	
ACCESS: 6 a.m.–11 p.m. year-round	

cutoff trail that would take 2.8 miles off your Blue Trail hike. Stay right and hike the southwestern portion of the Blue Trail, which is the most rugged section of the entire trail. The course zigs and zags with hairpins and rises and falls with ridges and kettles. The surface is full of tree roots, loose rocks, and exposed boulders. Some areas show plastic mesh or rubber water dams to help combat trail erosion.

This 2.9-mile segment starts south and then heads west in a bulge before it curves south and around back east. From there, it turns north to reconnect to the rest of the trail system, forming what looks roughly like a boot on the map. At the juncture, go right. Left is the Green Trail, the cutoff segment for this boot loop. You could go a few paces in this direction to find a trail to the north that would take you back to the Red Trail, where you could go right and find your way back to the trailhead for a total distance of 0.8 mile.

From the juncture, you have 2.6 miles left. Start downhill through pine forest, and then head straight across a small open field. The trail takes another big southerly loop, this time through slightly milder, though nevertheless challenging, terrain. As you make the return toward the north, the woods thin a bit and offer some sky above, and you pass through areas of brush and prairie. There's a bit of zigzagging and climbing to the trail in the last mile or so. The first juncture you come to is the Red Loop coming from the left. Go straight and the next right is the exit 0.1 mile to the lot.

Nearby Activities

Stop in at the LaGrange General Store, Café, and Deli (262-495-8600, **backyardbikes. com**) on US 12. Besides good sandwiches and something to drink, the place offers bicycle rentals and repairs.

Kettle Moraine State Forest: John Muir Trail

Young Road

Bluff Road

To
Emma Carlin
Trails (5.5 miles)

Bluff Road

Bluff Road

Duffin Road

CR H

*pioneer
lime kiln*

Nordic
Trails

Ice Age
National
Scenic Trail

P

?

KETTLE
MORAINE
STATE
FOREST

Greening Road

CR H

Duffin Road

To
67 43

12

Duffin Road

12

N

| 0 | 0.2 | 0.4 | 0.6 mile |

| 0 | 0.2 | 0.4 | 0.6 kilometer |

GPS COORDINATES AND DIRECTIONS

N42° 49' 12.30" W88° 36' 12.41"

From its intersection with US 12/18, go south 20.8 miles on I-39/90 to Exit 163 for Milton/Edgerton. Take WI 59 east (right at the end of the ramp) 2.8 miles to County Road N. Continue on CR N for 10.8 miles, until it becomes Walworth Avenue outside Whitewater. Turn right on US 12 and follow it 9.2 miles to La Grange. Turn left (north) on CR H, and go 1.6 miles to the John Muir Trail park entrance on the left. The trailhead is at the southwest corner of the parking lot near a map board kiosk.

57 Kettle Moraine State Forest: Lapham Peak Unit

The view from the observation tower on Lapham Peak

In Brief

Climb a tower at the highest peak in Waukesha County and be prepared to work as you hike the glacial roller coaster around this park that features a kettle moraine.

Description

Lapham Peak is named for Increase A. Lapham, a scientist and naturalist who came to Wisconsin in 1836 and wrote much about the state's wildlife and geology. Combined, there are 17 miles of loop trails here. The easiest trails are the Purple and Green loops. The course mapped out here is a loop of the entire park, primarily following the Black Loop, which has some rather strenuous up-and-down climbs. The asphalt Plantation Trail is wheelchair-accessible.

Begin from Parking Lot 9. The trailhead is not clearly marked, but look beyond the trail kiosk for a wide stretch of mowed trail—just to the left of the paved trail—with an arrow going away from you. Go straight to the woods. The trail goes up steeply on packed dirt into pine forest. At 0.2 mile, you pass a bench to the right. You find benches at nearly all trail junctures, in fact. Downhill to the right is a cutoff to the Plantation Trail, but follow the trail signs with a black circle on them. The trail continues with pine to the right and oak and maple to the left. At 0.1 mile is a trail to the butterfly garden just outside the woods here. Go straight another 0.2 mile to another trail juncture. The easy trail goes left here, and there is a map board.

LENGTH & CONFIGURATION: 6.9-mile loop	**MAPS:** USGS *Oconomowoc East;* at park office; map boards at trail junctures; **dnr.state.wi.us**
DIFFICULTY: Moderate to difficult	**WHEELCHAIR ACCESSIBILITY:** A separate 1.8-mile paved nature trail and a viewing platform near the observation tower
SCENERY: Mixed forest, prairie, kettle moraine, high-point overlook	
EXPOSURE: Mostly shaded	**FACILITIES:** Restrooms, water, park office
TRAFFIC: Light	
TRAIL SURFACE: Packed dirt, grass, some crushed rock	**CONTACT: dnr.wi.gov/topic/parks/ name/lapham,** 262-646-3025
HIKING TIME: 3 hours	**COMMENTS:** Dogs allowed. There is a state park vehicle registration fee ($7 daily, $25 annual for vehicles with WI plates; $10 daily, $35 annual for out-of-state plates).
DRIVING DISTANCE: 46 miles east from the I-39/94 interchange	
ACCESS: 7 a.m.–9 p.m. (10 p.m. in winter)	

A hard right takes you uphill to parking, and a soft right heads downhill. Watch for your trail symbol on the posts. The trail is shaded by oak-hickory forest, and the terrain rolls a lot.

You will cross the Ice Age Trail (IAT) 0.2 mile later, which goes left to right. The observation tower is to the right here, if you prefer to take the more rugged IAT. Regardless, the trail curves around to the right and brings you within a few feet of the IAT, where you find a spur trail. Take this and go left up some steps to the clearing where you can climb the 45-foot tower for some amazing views.

Return to the main path via the steps. You come to a trail juncture at "Stairway to Heaven." Stay straight and pass under some power lines where you come to The Big Slide. This path descends steeply and curves right where you find a cutoff heading up and back to the left if you want to skip the Green Loop/Meadow Trail. Stay right and hike another 0.1 mile before crossing the Ice Age Trail once again. To the right is the campsite for that trail and beyond that the tower again. Enter a clearing at 0.2 mile and go right. The trail to the left cuts off the meadow.

Another 0.1 mile brings you into the woods, and on your left you find American Indian marker trees, which look like bent elbows. There is an accompanying storyboard for them and another map board. Another cutoff trail goes left, but stay straight. This is Two Tier Trail, and the path goes up in two steep climbs for the next 800 feet. The trail forks at the top as you continue left. The park road is out to the right. Another 0.2 mile brings you to the other end of the last cutoff trail, and you continue out into an open field 0.2 mile after that.

This segment follows around prairie on mowed-grass paths. Stay on the main trail and don't take spur trails off to the right as they lead out of the trail system or to parking. The first spur to the left just 100 feet into the meadow cuts off the loop. Otherwise, it is

Kettle Moraine State Forest: Lapham Peak Unit

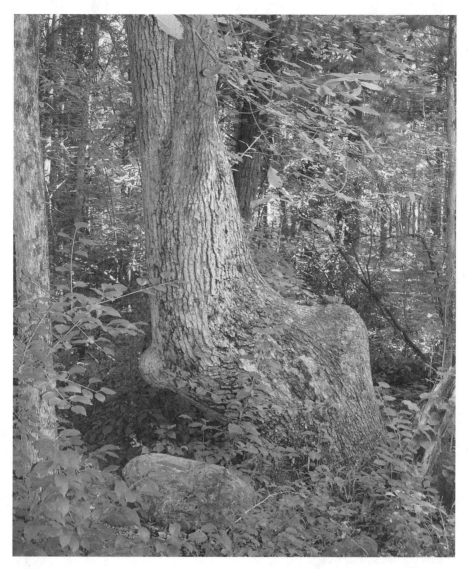

An American Indian marker tree

0.5 mile around to the other end and back into the woods where the cutoff trail rejoins the main trail. You will pass the Evergreen Grove picnic area and parking, where there are toilets and water.

When the trail comes back around to the woods, go right into the shade along some pines with oak savanna to your right. Pass the other end of a previous cutoff trail on your left at 400 feet. Go right as the trail takes a little elbow deep to the right along the edge of prairie, with oak savanna still to the right. Cross the IAT, which leads right to a pond overlook 1.25 miles to Menahbim Spring.

Crossing the IAT brings you to South Field. Follow along a rock wall to your right. Then the trail goes left along a long row of cedars. The path enters the woods once again, and you come to a trail map and juncture. To the left is part of the Green Loop. Go straight to a steep climb at South Hill, bringing you to another juncture. Stay right here. It's another 0.5 mile with a bit of climbing, and then you come to a bench. Another 300 feet brings you across a ski trail where there's another map board. Go straight. The trail dips down another 0.1 mile to another map board. The trail from the left is the end of the Stairway to Heaven trail, which came directly from the tower area. Keep going past this, and you pass Target Tree after another 0.2 mile.

At 0.2 mile, you come to another juncture. The black trail goes left here and enters a short loop of some of the more challenging short climbs of the trail. But to the right is Pete's Pass, which offers a view of a kettle moraine. I recommend going right here, which is the only time you part from the Black Loop. (This is a part of the Blue Trail). Alternatively, you could have a peek and come back for the challenge.

Pete's Pass ends 0.2 mile later, passing the kettle moraine on the right. The Black Loop joins again from the left, and the IAT crosses just a few steps after that. Just 250 feet later is yet another juncture with a trail map. Left is the easy Purple Trail coming from where you began your hike near the butterfly garden. Go right and, at 0.1 mile, find a map board and the Purple Trail heading left into prairie. Continue right and down into woods. At 0.2 mile, you pass the remains of a settler's cabin to your left. The trail continues along the top of a ridge with oak forest, and 300 feet later, gives you another option. Left is a cutoff that would take you 0.4 mile back to the trailhead bearing right at the first intersection along its length. Stay right on the Black Loop and face the steepest climb of the hike. Pass along Rock Ridge and cross a ravine to the left. The first juncture is at 0.6 mile. Go left on The Wimp's Trail to cut off the steepest climb. Go right to face The Wall. It's steep, but only about 200 feet long. The trail loops back around and comes to the end of the 400-foot Wimp's Trail cutoff 0.3 mile later.

The trail continues 0.3 mile to a juncture. Go straight to go out to the parking lot. Go right to wrap around a small scenic pond before coming back around and out alongside a shelter house. Follow the park road up to the parking lot where you began.

Nearby Activities

Nearby Delafield (**delafield-wi.org**) offers a historic downtown area and a variety of shops and boutiques.

GPS COORDINATES AND DIRECTIONS

N43° 02' 22.78" W88° 23' 33.34"

From the interchange of I-39/94, drive east 45.2 miles to Exit 285 to County Road C. Turn right (south) on CR C and drive 0.8 mile to the park entrance on the left. Follow the park road 0.7 mile to the Homestead Hollow parking area on the left. The trailhead is to the right of the restrooms behind the trail map kiosk.

58 Kettle Moraine State Forest: Nordic Trails

PHOTO: Preamtip Satasuk

A doubletrack through pine plantation on the Nordic Trails

In Brief

A web of ski trails offers many miles and combinations of treks over moraines and around kettles with the option for a serious workout.

Description

This collection of cross-country ski trails makes for several great hiking courses. The routes are color-coded and often overlap with each other to offer a variety of hike lengths. Options are many, from the half-mile Brown Trail to the 3.6-mile Green Trail. But the mother of them all is the 9-plus-mile outer loop Blue Trail, which manages to take in

LENGTH & CONFIGURATION: Up to 9.1 miles; loop	**ACCESS:** 6 a.m.–11 p.m. year-round
DIFFICULTY: Difficult due to length and frequent steep climbs; shorter easy options available	**MAPS:** USGS *Little Prairie;* at park office; posted at trail junctures
	WHEELCHAIR ACCESSIBILITY: None
SCENERY: Rich hardwood and pine forests, prairie, glacial rock formations	**FACILITIES:** Water, restrooms, picnic tables, grills and shelters
EXPOSURE: Mixed	**CONTACT:** dnr.wi.gov/topic/parks/name/kms/trails.html, 262-594-6200; Kettle Moraine Hiking Club: **kmhiking-club.webs.com**
TRAFFIC: Light to medium	
TRAIL SURFACE: Packed dirt, sand and scattered rock, mowed grass	**COMMENTS:** All vehicles require a park sticker ($7 daily, $25 annual for vehicles with WI plates). No hiking allowed when snow is on the ground. For trail conditions call 262-594-6202.
HIKING TIME: 4 hours	
DRIVING DISTANCE: 45.2 miles from the juncture of I-39/90 and US 12/18	

the entire variety of terrain and make you work for it. Along its route, there are cutoff options if you change your mind. All trails have clear mileage markers throughout.

The terrain, like much of the terrain in Kettle Moraine State Forest, is characterized by glacial deposits from the last round of the Ice Age. Abundant forest and some patches of prairie have reclaimed the lands, but the rolling trail reflects the various piles of till beneath.

To the west of the parking lot are two trailheads: The first is actually the return trail for skiers of the Red, Orange, Green, and Brown Trails. Skiers need to work through the park in a clockwise direction, but hikers can go as they please. The next trailhead, just north of the return trail, is where this hike begins. So follow the edge of the woods left behind the shelter, and the trail enters the woods on a crushed-stone surface that gives way to patches of grass and packed dirt.

At a quarter mile, the trail slopes down to the right through oaks and, soon after, more steeply on loose gravel. It comes back up and goes through a narrow corridor of prairie with abundant wildflowers and, in summer, many butterflies. Just past the 0.5-mile mark you'll come to a trail juncture. Go left to stay on the Blue Trail. This 1.8-mile loop will return to this juncture, coming from the trail straight ahead. Along the way, you will descend into pine plantation and, at the farthest point—the 1.5-mile mark—find a spur trail that connects to the nearby Ice Age Trail to the west. Cross two patches of prairie and you are back at this juncture. Go left (east) and pass the 2.5-mile marker.

In another 0.1 mile the trail splits; the shorter trails head to the right into an interior loop, but the Blue Trail goes left, climbing gradually through open terrain granting views as you gain elevation on this bluff. Just past the 3-mile mark, you are on top of the park with views of the surrounding tree-covered ridges. The trees close in again soon after, and at 3.4 miles is another juncture. Straight across the Orange Trail could lead you back

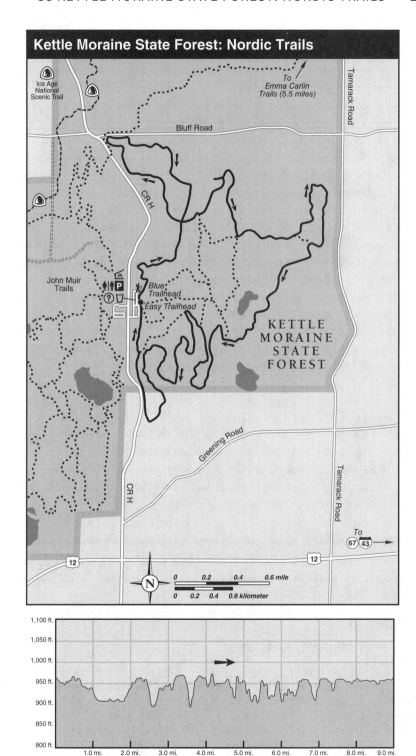

Kettle Moraine State Forest: Nordic Trails

Ice Age National Scenic Trail

Tamarack Road

To Emma Carlin Trails (5.5 miles)

Bluff Road

CR H

John Muir Trails

Blue Trailhead

Easy Trailhead

KETTLE MORAINE STATE FOREST

Greening Road

Tamarack Road

CR H

To 67 43

12

12

0   0.2   0.4   0.6 mile
0   0.2   0.4   0.6 kilometer

N

1,100 ft.
1,050 ft.
1,000 ft.
950 ft.
900 ft.
850 ft.
800 ft.

1.0 mi.   2.0 mi.   3.0 mi.   4.0 mi.   5.0 mi.   6.0 mi.   7.0 mi.   8.0 mi.   9.0 mi.

to the lot in just over a mile. The Green and Orange enter from the right (west) here, but you go left (east) on the Blue and Green Trails, descending through forest dominated by oaks and skirting a depression in the forest floor on the right, a kettle moraine. Through the trees on the left, depending on foliage, you may also see some kettle ponds.

Pass a bench on the right at 3.8 miles and 100 feet later is the next trail juncture. Green goes to the right, but stay straight to follow a 0.9-mile northerly loop of the Blue through pine-dominated woods. The Green Trail here would cut 0.8 mile off the hike. The Blue Trail turns back south at 4.2 miles, passing a service road on the left and finally reconnecting to the Green at 4.7 miles; go left.

The trail begins to show deep dips and steep climbs as it passes over short rolling terrain. Climbs are short, maybe 50 feet at a go, and benches are frequent. On the right, you can see another kettle pool through the trees. Pass the 5.5-mile marker and you'll soon come to a juncture where the Green Trail leaves to the right. Following this would put you just about a mile from the parking lot on easier trails; from here, the Blue Trail shows some of its hardest hiking, which is only to say a lot of up and down in short bursts.

Continue, past the 6-mile mark, and come to the longest of the dips, a stretch of about 75 feet down and up. Just past here, look for the deep kettles on either side of the trail as the path straddles the ridge between them. At 6.6 miles, the Purple and White Trails come straight at you. Stay on the Blue and follow to the left. Purple and White join the route here, but, at the next juncture, Purple goes straight, while you head left on the Blue and White Trails. Pass the 1-mile marker of the White and you have 2.2 miles left.

The trail has already become gentler and even flat in many places, with a mix of shade and open skies. Pass the 8.5-mile marker and the trail turns north and runs parallel to CR H—the home stretch. Pass a dip in the trail at 8.8 miles and it brings you up to a juncture where the Purple Trail connects from the right. Go left here and follow flat terrain and a straight bit through some pine before rounding one last bend to the left as you come upon the park facilities. You'll pass the start of the Purple, White, and Brown Trails on your right just before you reach the picnic area and parking lot.

Nearby Activities

The Turner Museum, operated by the Palmyra Historical Society, features historic artifacts and exhibits about Palmyra's past. A gift shop is also located at the museum. Stop in at 112 North Third St. in Palmyra, or call 262-495-2412.

GPS COORDINATES AND DIRECTIONS
N42° 49' 18.97" W88° 36' 1.10"

From its intersection with US 12/18, go south 20.8 miles on I-39/90 to Exit 163 for Milton/Edgerton. Take WI 59 east (right at the end of the ramp) 2.8 miles to County Road N for 10.8 miles where it becomes Walworth Avenue outside Whitewater. Turn right on US 12 and follow it 9.2 miles to La Grange. Go left (north) on CR H 1.6 miles to the Nordic Trail park entrance on the right, opposite John Muir Trail. The trailhead is behind the shelter on the northeast side of the parking lot.

59 Kettle Moraine State Forest: Scuppernong Trail

A trail through a pine plantation

In Brief

Rolling hills through pine forest and a view for miles from a scenic overlook are the highlights of this hike through some of southeastern Wisconsin's finest post-glacier terrain.

Description

The short climbs over rolling terrain and a generally good trail surface make this trail popular with cross-country runners. The trail outlined here follows the Green Loop, the outermost and longest loop in this section of the forest. On the black-and-white maps from the park office, all trails appear the same, but the overlap can be clarified against the color-coded map boards at trail junctures.

From the trailhead, the path turns left just inside the trees. A park access road continues straight from here. The first trail juncture is 200 feet farther along, and this is where the loop will return. Go right and follow a sandy lane strewn with pine needles. The lane goes straight through an orderly pine plantation 0.1 mile, where it bends left a little and leaves orderly pines for scattered spruces for a moment before heading back into pine plantation.

Another 0.15 mile later, hardwoods enter the mix, though pine is still the dominant species and the trail doesn't offer much shade. After 0.15 mile, you pass a bench, and then the rolling terrain really starts offering more of a workout than the flat stretch at the beginning.

LENGTH & CONFIGURATION: 5.4-mile loop	**MAPS:** USGS *Eagle;* in map box at park office; posted at trail junctures
DIFFICULTY: Easy to moderate	**FACILITIES:** Restrooms, water, picnic tables, grills
SCENERY: Pine forest, hardwood forest, overlooks	**CONTACT: dnr.wi.gov/topic/parks/ name/kms/trails.html,** 262-594-6200
EXPOSURE: Mostly shaded	**COMMENTS:** Leashed dogs allowed. No hiking or dogs when snow is present. All vehicles require a park sticker ($7 daily, $25 annual for vehicles with WI plates). Trail activities other than hiking incur a $4 daily fee ($20 annual). The small park office is typically closed, but you can self-register there. Parts of the park are open to gun hunting; during deer season at the end of November, wear bright clothing, especially blaze orange. Call 262-594-6200 to find out if the hunt is on.
TRAFFIC: Light to moderate	
TRAIL SURFACE: Packed dirt, sand, crushed rock, some tree roots and stones, some grass	
HIKING TIME: 1.5–2 hours	
DRIVING DISTANCE: 52 miles east of the I-39/94 interchange	
ACCESS: 6 a.m.–11 p.m. year-round	

From the bench to the next juncture is 0.25 mile. If you choose to go straight, it is the easy Red Loop that offers an inner loop back to the parking lot for a total of 2.3 miles. A hard right turn takes you down the short trail to D. J. Mackie group picnic area, where there is also water and parking. Take the soft right on the Green/Orange loops. The forest offers an abundance of chipmunks and squirrels, and you are likely to see a deer or two the farther you are from the parking areas and the open pine plantation. Sand gives way to a lot more scattered rock, and the up and down climbs are slightly steeper and more frequent from this point.

From this juncture, at 0.75 mile, cross the Ice Age National Scenic Trail (IAT) on your right. Before you is a map board with #6 on it. To the left is the IAT and a bench. The IAT is marked with yellow patches on trees and trail posts and it is a narrow footpath of packed dirt. You have the option to go left here on the IAT, which would present a bit more rugged hiking and take 1.3 miles off the Green Loop. Otherwise, continue right on the Green Loop.

Another 0.6 mile takes you to the edge of a small clearing. The trail bends around left here, passing a bench on the left, and then continues down old fire lanes. The trail goes south 0.2 mile, passing a picnic table and fire pit amid pine and brush on your right. Occasionally, turkey vultures roost here, so step softly and scan the branches. The trail bends right, and on your left you find the return path for the Orange Loop. Take this to cut your hike down to 4.2 miles.

There is a map board labeled #9 and a bench. Go right down a 0.3-mile corridor heading back north under pine and on the other side of those fire pits you just passed. Climb a short incline at the end to reach Point #10. Across this small field is a road into Pinewoods Campground, where you can find water and toilets. Go left, with the prairie on your right and woods on your left. The trail reenters the pines. You find some fern,

Kettle Moraine State Forest: Scuppernong Trail

wildflowers, and the occasional oak tree. Raspberries can be found here in midsummer during a good year. From Point #10, it's 0.5 mile through the pine until you cross the IAT once again. Continue straight as the canopy opens up. The trail curves right and downhill through short pines on a grassy trail 0.4 mile until the next juncture and map board at Point #14.

The left path is the return on the Orange Loop and backward on the Red Loop. Go right on crushed rock into shade. About 300 feet along, you come to the Observation Loop, a short 0.4-mile lollipop to the right. It's 0.1 mile to the fork where you go right and follow the loop as it becomes a bit narrower and more rugged with roots and rocks. Another 0.2 mile from the fork is an overlook with a couple of benches and the valley beyond. What you see is a glacial sand plain and a couple of small lakes, as well as a long view to the horizon.

Return to the head of the Observation Loop and continue right on the main trail. At 0.25 mile, you come to a wide intersection with a map board. Straight ahead are the Red and Orange loops. Go right on the Green Loop where a sign indicates this is the hardest trail for skiers. This jagged portion of the loop heads west, passing a scenic overlook under oak trees. These will be the steepest climbs, and the descents can be slippery in wet weather. The Red Loop, which parts left from the Orange Loop 0.15 mile down the trail, would bypass the steepest parts.

On the Green Loop you find a scenic overlook at 0.2 mile. From there, the trail takes a sharp left and heads downhill. Another 0.25 mile takes you up another hill and then down a 200-foot, moderately steep decline. You start to see pine once again on your left. Pass another bench at 0.15 mile and yet another 0.1 mile after that, where there is also a map board where the Orange Loop comes in from the left. After a bend in the trail, you come to a 50-foot, steep and uneven descent. Be cautious of loose rock. Another 75 feet later is a similar ramp with tree roots and potentially slippery mud. You reach pine plantation for the final 0.2 mile to the end of the trail. Just before you arrive there, you see the Red Loop joining from the left, then the beginning of the loop going left just after that. Head straight out and follow the bend to the right to return to the trailhead.

Nearby Activities

The State Forest Visitor Center (262-594-6200) is on WI 59, 3 miles west of Eagle. Scuppernong Springs is a 1.5-mile, self-guided nature trail nearby. Pick up a booklet at the trailhead.

GPS COORDINATES AND DIRECTIONS
N42° 56' 26.82" W88° 27' 41.87"

From where I-94 departs from I-39 and heads east toward Milwaukee, take I-94 for 41.2 miles to WI 67. Go south 9.9 miles to County Road ZZ, turn left, and go 0.4 mile to the park entrance. The trailhead is at the north corner of the lot.

60 Lake Kegonsa State Park

Wetlands near Williams Bay

In Brief

This lakeside park offers several short hikes or one long one that takes in varying landscape that includes restored prairie, a pine plantation, oak forest, and a marsh. Afterward, go for a swim.

Description

This park was once part of a great river valley that was here more than a million years ago. The last of the glaciers passed over this area; where they stopped, they left a line of glacial deposit called a terminal moraine, located today just a few miles south of Lake Kegonsa. The meltwater flowing from the shrinking glaciers filled some of the former river valley with sand, gravel, and large boulders, forming dams in some places and raising the base significantly. The result is the chain of four lakes in the Madison area.

The park has several trails that can be combined, as they are here, to make a long hike through a variety of terrain. If you just want to take White Oak Nature Trail and Prairie Trail, you should take the first right after the park office for trail parking. For the complete hike, go to the beach parking area and find the paved walkway at the corner of the lot near the changing rooms.

Pass the small beach area on your right. The trail takes you through a pleasant picnic area along the lakeshore. Four hundred feet down the path, you'll pass a gate in a wooden fence and then the pet swim area on your right. The trail crosses a culvert that connects

LENGTH & CONFIGURATION:
5.3 miles of multiple loops

DIFFICULTY: Easy

SCENERY: Prairie, marsh, forest, lakeshore

EXPOSURE: Mostly sun

TRAFFIC: Light

TRAIL SURFACE: Mostly cut grass or packed limestone, some dirt, asphalt

HIKING TIME: 2.5–3 hours

DRIVING DISTANCE: 8.5 miles south from the intersection of US 12/18 and Interstate 39

ACCESS: 6 a.m.–11 p.m. year-round

MAPS: USGS *Stoughton;* on the DNR website and at park office

WHEELCHAIR ACCESSIBILITY:
Yes, on Lakeshore Trail, Prairie Trail, and boardwalk; accessible picnic tables, restrooms, and a railing for lake entry at the beach

FACILITIES: Restrooms, picnic areas with grills, campground, changing rooms, vending machines, pay phones, water

CONTACT: dnr.wi.gov/topic/parks/ name/lakekegonsa, 608-873-9695

COMMENTS: Leashed dogs allowed; pet swim area. A self-guided hike through the forest includes a booklet available at the office or White Oak trailhead. All vehicles require a park sticker ($7 daily, $25 annual for vehicles with WI plates). The park participates in the Junior Ranger/Wisconsin Explorer program (see Preface, page 8).

the marshy area to your left to the lake on your right and then goes under tall cottonwoods as it loops through the mowed area past benches and a small dock before arriving at another parking area. Stay left here and walk past the pit toilets and through the parking lot to the park road. Just out of the parking lot, look for a yellow sign on the right side of the road that marks the trail.

This little half loop ventures through mixed forest for 750 feet before rejoining the road. At the end of this segment is the Williams Knoll picnic area, where you can still see the old foundation of the carriage house of John Williams, who once owned much of the park land when he came to Wisconsin in the 19th century.

Follow the park road now to the right. Just past the parking lot on the left is a trail entrance to the Oak Knoll Trail, which begins with prairie. The trail left heads straight back to the pet swim area. Go right here along the park road through a nicely restored prairie full of native species of wildflowers. At the next small parking lot, go left following the lot's edge and follow the trail around to where it connects to a left-to-right trail along the edge of the trees. Left takes you back in a small prairie loop; go right along the edge of an oak and hickory forest, with the prairie now to your right.

The trail cuts through the woods across a mowed circle and reemerges amid coneflowers, bergamot, black-eyed Susans, and Queen Anne's lace. Here is another juncture-with a trail leading right to the road. Go left, with the prairie on your right, and look for Turk's-cap lilies through here.

After only 400 feet, you are back into woods with aspen and black walnut until, another 400 feet later, you find that trail back to the pet exercise area. It's 800 feet back to the wooden fence by the beach, and halfway there you cross a bridge that offers a very

A bridge crosses a narrow marshy area.

nice view of the marsh on both sides. Return to the parking area and take a stroll down the short boardwalk to the right to look for waterfowl in the marsh.

Continuing from the end of the boardwalk, walk along the right side of the lot heading north. To your right, the marsh is visible in early spring or after the leaves are gone in fall. You'll come to a second parking lot; at the end of the grassy median in that lot, look for a trail sign.

Walk 700 feet through more prairie to a trail juncture. The path on the left crosses the road to Bluebird Trail; save this for the end if you'd like. Go right and cross the park road. On the other side is a metal gate. Go around the gate and again cross a road, Williams Point Drive. Cross at an angle to a sign that reads TRAIL TO CAMPGROUND. Walk through a short corridor of foliage and then into open prairie. The trail forks here. To the right are the campgrounds. Go left on an exposed path, with prairie on your right and shrubs to the left.

At 900 feet, go right at the trail juncture, crossing the prairie and then bearing left at the opposite side. This is the closest point to the park office, and you'll pass a small spur trail that would let you out there. Continue until the next place to cross the park road. On the other side, the trail goes left or right. Stay right following the curve of crushed limestone. This is the Prairie Trail and is wheelchair accessible. Look for compass flowers in the field. At the next juncture, go right into woods. Here there is a sign for identifying wildflowers. Leadplant, spiderwort, purple prairie clover, butterfly milkweed, and various grasses reside here, and this sign helps you find them.

It's only 100 feet to the head of the White Oak Nature Trail and its 14 numbered stations that correspond to the self-guided nature tour booklet. There should be some at the trailhead if you didn't pick one up at the park office. A playground and flush toilets are here next to the parking lot.

White Oak Nature Trail is a 1.2-mile loop with packed-dirt surface and a lot of tree roots. The rise and fall of the land make this more strenuous than the prairie segments but nothing more than moderate. Tall oaks and various other trees provide plenty of shade. Look for black raspberries here in late June. Going right, you encounter American Indian ceremonial mounds at 0.3 mile, where the trail curves left within the park boundaries. Another 0.4 mile brings you to the entrance of the Pine Plantation. Go right here and have a look at the red needle carpet and the most fragrant part of the forest. Back on the main trail, pass more mounds to the right. Then the trail climbs back up to the trailhead once again, where there's a bench if you need a break.

From White Oak Nature Trail, go right and take a crushed-limestone trail to your right that passes through a fire pit area and out into the prairie again. Go right at the trail juncture as the path takes you 0.3 mile south across the edge of the prairie to the next juncture. To the left is a cutoff for the Prairie Trail. Instead, go right on the group camping trail, a 0.6-mile loop around more prairie. As the trail curves and heads back, it passes through a shaded corridor of locust trees before coming back into the open at a baseball diamond to the left of the trail.

The trail rejoins the Prairie Trail as you continue with it to the right until you come once again to a crossing of the park road. On the other side, pick up a trail that goes left along the road or right into the prairie. Take that right path and follow it straight across the prairie 0.3 mile to where it comes once again to where you started into the fields. Go right here through the brush and cross the two park roads to arrive at a sign that reads TRAIL TO BEACH. Here you have the option of going right across the parking lot entry road to hike along a small hill covered with wildflowers on a 0.3-mile loop that is Bluebird Trail. On this trail, you immediately come to a fork. Going left up the hill, you come to another juncture. Go right. The trail left leads to a picnic area on top of the hill, where there are pit toilets and water. As the loop comes back around, you see an exit to the road on your left as the trail continues right through a stand of aspens. Soon you are back where you started, and you can cross the road to the Trail to Beach and head right back to the parking area.

Nearby Activities

Cinema Café at 124 West Main St. in nearby Stoughton combines big-screen movies with homemade pizza served while you enjoy the show. Call 608-873-7484 or go to **stoughton-cinemacafe.com** to find out what's playing.

GPS COORDINATES AND DIRECTIONS
N42° 58' 22.39" W89° 13' 49.18"

From its intersection with US 12/18, drive south 5.2 miles on I-39 to the County Road N exit. Turn right (south) and at 0.6 mile turn right on Koshkonong Road, taking it 1.7 miles to its end at Door Creek Road. Go left 1 mile to the park entrance on your right. After checking in at the main office, follow the park road as it curves back around under an overpass, and then take the second right to beach parking. The trail begins at the sidewalk near the beach.

Appendix A: Hiking Stores

Fontana Sports

Downtown
  216 North Henry St.
  Madison, WI 53703
  608-257-5043
  fontanasports.com

West Madison
  231 Junction Road
  Madison, WI 53717
  608-833-9191

Gander Mountain
  6199 East Metro Drive
  De Forest, WI 53532
  608-242-9532
  gandermountain.com

REI
  7483 West Towne Way
  Madison, WI 53719
  608-833-6680
  rei.com

The Shoe Box
  US 14 (at the stoplight in Black Earth)
  Black Earth, WI 53515
  608-767-3447
  theshoebox.com

Baraboo Outlet Store
  141 Third Ave.
  Baraboo, WI 53913
  608-356-1224
  theshoebox.com

Appendix B: Map Stores

Eagle Eye Maps

50 Merlham Drive
Madison, WI 53705
608-233-9037
eagleeyemaps.com

Ice Age Trail Alliance

2110 Main St.
Cross Plains, WI 53528
800-227-0046
iceagetrail.org (Click: Store)

Mapping Specialists, Ltd.

3000 Cahill Main, Suite 220
Fitchburg, WI 53711
608-274-4004
mappingspecialists.com

Wisconsin Geological and Natural History Survey

3817 Mineral Point Road
Madison, WI 53705
608-263-7389
wisconsingeologicalsurvey.org

Appendix C: Hiking Clubs

Meetup.com hosts various grass-roots hiking groups, which are free to join and subscribe to, including Madison Area Women's Outdoor Network, Madison Outdoor Network, Southern Wisconsin Day Hiking, Madison LGBT Outdoor Group, and Wisconsin Outdoor Group. Connect online at **hiking.meetup.com/cities/us/wi/madison** to see them all and to find planned events.

Ice Age Trail Alliance
2110 Main St.
Cross Plains, WI 53528
800-227-0046
.iceagetrail.org

The Ice Age Trail Alliance is a great resource for the Ice Age Trail and produces its own complete trail guide and a companion Ice Age Trail Atlas. Additionally, the alliance is supported by 21 volunteer chapters, which help build and maintain various segments throughout the trail. These chapters have occasional hiking and volunteer work events. Additionally, many of them have created certificates and honors for hikers who complete that chapter's combined trail segments. Check each chapter's website for phone numbers or to download each program brochure.

Baraboo Hills Chapter
baraboohills.iceagetrail.org

Dane County Chapter
dane.iceagetrail.org

Lodi Valley Chapter
lodivalley.iceagetrail.org

Rock County Chapter
rock.iceagetrail.org

Walworth/Jefferson County Chapter
walworthjefferson.iceagetrail.org

John Muir Chapter Sierra Club
222 South Hamilton St., #1
Madison, WI 53703
608-256-0565
wisconsin.sierraclub.org

Kettle Moraine Hiking Club
kmhikingclub.webs.com
kmhikingclub@gmail.com

Wisconsin Hoofers Outing Club
800 Langdon St.
Madison, WI 53706
608-262-1630
hooferouting.org

Index

About the Author

KEVIN REVOLINSKI'S love for the outdoors came from frequent childhood fishing trips and hikes with his father in the woods of northern Wisconsin. He is the author of more than a dozen books, including *The Yogurt Man Cometh: Tales of an American Teacher in Turkey, Wisconsin's Best Beer Guide: A Travel Companion* (also Michigan and Minnesota versions), and *Backroads and Byways of Wisconsin,* and is coauthor of *Best Tent Camping: Wisconsin.* He has written for Rough Guides guidebooks, and his articles and photography have appeared in a variety of publications, including *The New York Times, Chicago Tribune, Wisconsin Trails,* and the *Miami Herald.* He has lived abroad in several places, including Turkey, Italy, Guatemala, Panama, and Thailand, but currently makes camp back in the homeland in Madison, Wisconsin. Check out his website at **themadtraveleronline.com** and his blog **revtravel.com.**

PHOTO: Preamtip Satasuk

DEAR CUSTOMERS AND FRIENDS,

SUPPORTING YOUR INTEREST IN OUTDOOR ADVENTURE, travel, and an active lifestyle is central to our operations, from the authors we choose to the locations we detail to the way we design our books. Menasha Ridge Press was incorporated in 1982 by a group of veteran outdoorsmen and professional outfitters. For many years now, we've specialized in creating books that benefit the outdoors enthusiast.

Almost immediately, Menasha Ridge Press earned a reputation for revolutionizing outdoors- and travel-guidebook publishing. For such activities as canoeing, kayaking, hiking, backpacking, and mountain biking, we established new standards of quality that transformed the whole genre, resulting in outdoor-recreation guides of great sophistication and solid content. Menasha Ridge continues to be outdoor publishing's greatest innovator.

The folks at Menasha Ridge Press are as at home on a whitewater river or mountain trail as they are editing a manuscript. The books we build for you are the best they can be, because we're responding to your needs. Plus, we use and depend on them ourselves.

We look forward to seeing you on the river or the trail. If you'd like to contact us directly, join in at trekalong.com or visit us at menasharidge .com. We thank you for your interest in our books and the natural world around us all.

SAFE TRAVELS,

Bob Sehlinger

BOB SEHLINGER
PUBLISHER